MW00667953

Kristine A. Karlsen, PhD, APRN
Neonatal Nurse Practitioner
Author/Founder
National Program Director
The S.T.A.B.L.E. Program
Park City, Utah

Lloyd Y. Tani, MD
Technical Consulting Editor
Professor of Pediatrics
Director of Echocardiography
University of Utah and
Primary Children's Medical Center
Salt Lake City, Utah

Address correspondence to:
The S.T.A.B.L.E. Program
P.O. Box 980023
Park City, Utah 84098-0023 USA
Phone (435)-655-8171
www.stableprogram.org

ISBN: 0-9758559-0-5
ISBN 13: 978-0-9758559-0-4

Content Reviewers
Carl L. Bose, MD
Professor of Pediatrics
Chief, Division of Neonatal-Perinatal Medicine
University of North Carolina
Chapel Hill, North Carolina

Janet Craig, RN, MS, PNP
Pediatric Cardiology Nurse Practitioner
Primary Children's Medical Center
Salt Lake City, Utah

Laurale M. Cross, RNC, NNP
Neonatal Nurse Practitioner
Valley View Hospital
Glenwood Springs, Colorado

Vicki Greenland, RN, BSN
NICU Cardiac Resource Nurse
Primary Children's Medical Center
Salt Lake City, Utah

Tracy B. Karp, MS, RNC, NNP
Manager, Neonatal Nurse Practitioner Service
Primary Children's Medical Center
Salt Lake City, Utah

Linda M. Lambert, MSN, CFNP
Cardiothoracic Nurse Practitioner
Pediatric Cardiothoracic Surgery
Primary Children's Medical Center
Salt Lake City, Utah

CAPT Martin J. McCaffrey, MD
Specialty Advisor to the Navy Surgeon
General for Neonatology
Director Neonatal Intensive Care Unit
Naval Medical Center San Diego
San Diego, California

L. LuAnn Minich, MD
Pediatric Cardiology
Associate Professor of Pediatrics
University of Utah and
Primary Children's Medical Center
Salt Lake City, Utah

Luciana T. Young, MD
Pediatric Cardiology
Associate Professor of Pediatrics
University of Utah and
Primary Children's Medical Center
Salt Lake City, Utah

Beta Testers
Sandy Bellini, RNC, MS, NNP
Neonatology Associates
UMass-Memorial Health Care
Worcester, Massachusetts

Marion E. DeLand, RNC
Neonatal Nurse Educator
Sunnybrook and
Women's College Health Sciences Center
Toronto, Ontario, Canada

Webra Price-Douglas, PhD, CRNP, IBCLC
Neonatal Transport Coordinator
Maryland Regional Neonatal
Transport Program
Baltimore, Maryland

Kathryn Rudd, MSN, RNC
Level III Neonatal Intensive Care Unit
Staff Nurse
MetroHealth Medical Center
Cleveland, Ohio

Medical Illustrator
Marilou Kundmueller RN, BSN, MA,
Medical Illustration
Salt Lake City, Utah

Graphic Designer
Kristin Bernhisel-Osborn, MFA
Primary Children's Medical Center
Salt Lake City, Utah

Copy Editor
Heather Bennett
Hither & Yon
Salt Lake City, Utah

Endorsed by

March of Dimes
Saving babies, together
1.888.966.3222
marchofdimes.com

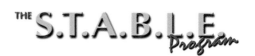

Improving Neonatal Outcomes — with Education

i

For Torbjorn, Annika and Solveig, whose support has sustained me through this creation,

and for all of the incredible neonatal healthcare providers I have had

the privilege to meet on my journey with S.T.A.B.L.E.

Your expert teaching and guidance will make a difference in the lives of many babies.

Contents

Physical Exam

Cyanotic CHD
Not ductal dependent

Cyanotic CHD
Ductal dependent for PBF

Left outflow tract CHD
Ductal dependent for SBF

S.T.A.B.L.E. Program

S.T.A.B.L.E.® – Cardiac Module

Sugar, Temperature, Airway, Blood Pressure, Lab Work, and Emotional Support

The S.T.A.B.L.E. Program is an educational program designed for all maternal/child health care providers (nurses, physicians, respiratory therapists, and pre-hospital providers) to address the pre-transport stabilization and post-resuscitation care of sick neonates. All information in the basic S.T.A.B.L.E. Program Learner Course applies to neonates with cardiac conditions. This module includes additional guidelines for neonates with severe congenital heart disease (CHD). We recommend that participants complete the S.T.A.B.L.E. Program Learner Course prior to reviewing this module. More information about the S.T.A.B.L.E. Program can be found at **www.stableprogram.org**.

Introduction

Each year, approximately 40,000 babies, or just under 1% of all babies born in the United States, are diagnosed with CHD. As many as one-third of these babies will be critically ill and require care by neonatal and cardiac experts in the first days to weeks of life. Depending on the type of heart problem, initial signs and symptoms may include tachypnea, cyanosis, and/or a heart murmur. With severe forms of CHD, there may be marked cyanosis, respiratory distress, and rapid progression to advanced states of shock. Prompt, effective care of neonates with CHD can reduce secondary organ damage, improve short and long-term outcomes, and reduce mortality.

> This instructional program is intended to provide only general guidelines for the assessment and stabilization of neonates with suspected congenital heart disease. Many neonatal illnesses and conditions are not discussed in this manual. You should consult neonatal and/or cardiac experts, or refer to additional educational materials, as needed, before treating any sick neonates. The content of the S.T.A.B.L.E. Program Cardiac Module should be reviewed and approved by appropriate policy committees before its principles and procedures are implemented at your institution.

Goals of this Module

1. Review the clinical presentation and initial stabilization of neonates with severe and/or life-threatening heart defects.

2. Provide the learner with information to improve their care of neonates with CHD.

Course Objectives

In completing this module, the learner will gain an increased understanding of the following concepts:

1. Physical assessment of neonates with suspected CHD;

2. Anatomic features, clinical presentation, and initial stabilization of neonates with CHD.

This manual has been designed to accompany the S.T.A.B.L.E. – Cardiac module PowerPoint® presentation. Part 1 will focus on the physical examination of neonates with suspected CHD; Part 2 will explore differentiation of cardiac from lung disease, and the presentation and stabilization of the most severe heart defects seen in neonates; and Part 3 will discuss adaptations to the basic S.T.A.B.L.E. program modules — **S**ugar, **T**emperature, **A**irway, **B**lood pressure, **L**ab work and **E**motional support — that are necessary to care for neonates with CHD.

Vital Signs – Respiratory Rate and Effort

Normal

Respiratory rate is 30 to 60 breaths per minute.

Breathing is not labored, with easy effort.

Abnormal

Tachypnea

A respiratory rate > 60 breaths per minute, without signs of respiratory distress (comfortably tachypneic), may be one of the first signs of cardiac disease.

Respiratory signs of severe congestive heart failure or shock

♥ Labored breathing

♥ Sternal and intercostal retractions

♥ Grunting

♥ Nasal flaring

Respiratory rate < 30

A slow respiratory rate, in association with labored breathing, may signal exhaustion. It may also represent a decrease in central respiratory drive because of narcotic depression, hypoxic ischemic encephalopathy, or other causes.

 Gasping is an ominous sign of impending cardiorespiratory arrest. If the infant is gasping, initiate emergency respiratory and cardiovascular resuscitative measures.

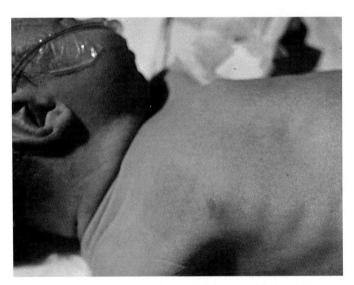

Figure 1.1. 36-week gestation infant with transient tachypnea of the newborn. Note the mild intercostal retractions.

Vital Signs – Heart Rate and Rhythm

Normal

The heart rate in the neonate is usually between 120 and 160 beats/minute, with a normal range of 80 and 200 beats/minute. Lower heart rates are usually seen at rest, whereas higher heart rates are seen when the infant is active or crying. When in deep sleep, some normal infants may have heart rates as low as 70 beats/minute.

Abnormal

Bradycardia

A heart rate < 70 beats/minute in a neonate usually represents pathologic bradycardia.

 Hypoxemia, hypotension, and acidosis depress the conduction system and may lead to bradycardia. Therefore any neonate with a heart rate < 100 should be assessed for signs of hemodynamic compromise or shock. If shock is detected, bradycardia indicates the neonate is in severe crisis.

Sinus bradycardia should be differentiated from complete heart block. In *sinus bradycardia*, a QRS complex follows each p wave (see figure 1.2). Underlying causes of sinus bradycardia include increased vagal tone, mechanical causes such as a central venous line located in the high right atrium, and apnea. In *complete heart block* the p wave is completely unrelated to the QRS complexes, indicating the atrial impulses are not conducted into the ventricle (see Figure 1.3). The ventricular (QRS) rate usually ranges from 45 to 80 beats/minute. An increased incidence is seen with maternal systemic lupus erythematosus and other connective tissue diseases. Neonates who present at birth with hydrops secondary to complete heart block are critically ill.

Tachycardia

Sinus tachycardia versus supraventricular tachycardia

Crying or agitated neonates occasionally have heart rates that reach 200–220 beats/minute, however a sustained heart rate greater than 180 beats/minute is abnormal.

Neonates in shock or congestive heart failure may have a sustained *sinus tachycardia*, with heart rates ranging between 180 and 220 beats/minute.

Neonates with *supraventricular tachycardia (SVT)* usually have sustained heart rates > 220 beats/minute. Most babies tolerate SVT and do not develop shock. The exception is the neonate who presents with hydrops or concurrent structural heart disease. The presence of shock should be determined by evaluating perfusion, pulses, presence of metabolic acidosis, blood pressure, respiratory compromise, and altered level of consciousness.

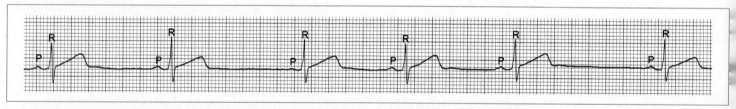

Figure 1.2. ECG of sinus bradycardia. The heart rate is 42 beats per minute. Note the QRS complex follows each p wave.

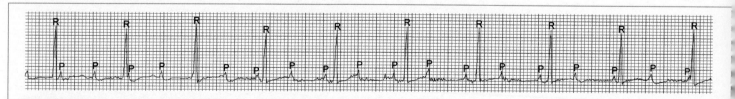

Figure 1.3. ECG of complete heart block. The atrial rate is 133 and the ventricular rate is 68. Note the p wave is unrelated to the QRS complex.

Vital Signs – Heart Rate and Rhythm

Treatment of Supraventricular Tachycardia (SVT)

Vagal maneuvers to stop SVT

Option one: Stimulate a gag.

Option two: Suction the nasopharynx.

Option three: Apply crushed ice to the nose and forehead area.

Procedure for performing the "icing" vagal maneuver

1. Place 1 cup of crushed ice in a plastic bag and cover the plastic bag with a thin cloth.

2. Start a rhythm strip.

3. Apply the ice bag to the nose and forehead area for approximately 15 seconds — or less if SVT stops.

4. It is not necessary to obstruct the airway with the ice bag.

5. Continue the rhythm strip through the "break" to normal sinus rhythm or, if SVT continues, for 1 minute.

6. When SVT stops, monitor the heart rate for conversion back to SVT.

7. If SVT continues, notify the pediatric cardiologist or neonatologist for further instructions.

- *This procedure is not recommended for neonates experiencing severe cardiac compromise or shock.*

- *If the neonate has a history of no response to ice, do not continue to attempt this maneuver. Proceed to adenosine administration.*

- *The application of ice may cause fatty tissue necrosis if the bag is applied over fatty tissue (cheeks) for a prolonged period of time (more than 15–20 seconds).*

- *Discard the ice bag after one application; refreezing the bag causes frost to form on it, increasing the probability that it will burn the neonate's face if reapplied.*

If the neonate is unstable or in shock, vagal maneuvers may be poorly tolerated and direct current (DC) cardioversion (usually 0.5 joules/kg) is the treatment of choice. If DC cardioversion is not available, then adenosine should be given to terminate SVT.

Adenosine (Adenocard®)

Adenosine is an antiarrhythmic agent used for the treatment of SVT. This drug restores normal sinus rhythm by slowing AV nodal conduction and interrupting its re-entry pathways.

Dose

1. Initial dose is 100 micrograms per kilogram (mcg/kg) **rapid IV push** over 1 to 2 seconds.

2. Follow the adenosine push with 2 to 3 ml of sterile normal saline flush.

3. If there is no response within 2 minutes, increase by 50 mcg/kg increments every 2 minutes until a maximum dose of 250 mcg/kg is given.

Weight (kg)		Dose (mcg)		Total dose (mcg)	Administer this amount
1	x	100	=	100	0.33 ml
1.5	x	100	=	150	0.5 ml
2	x	100	=	200	0.67 ml
2.5	x	100	=	250	0.83 ml
3	x	100	=	300	1 ml
3.5	x	100	=	350	1.17 ml
4	x	100	=	400	1.33 ml
4.5	x	100	=	450	1.5 ml
5	x	100	=	500	1.67 ml

Table 1.1. Adenosine Dosing by Infant's Weight

Preparing the medication

1. Use adenosine 3000 mcg/ml solution (3 mg/ml).

2. Dilute 1 ml of adenosine with 9 mls of sterile normal saline to yield a 300 mcg/ml solution (1:10 dilution).

Vital Signs – Heart Rate and Rhythm

Adverse reactions

Cardiovascular

Flushing, arrhythmias, chest pain, bradycardia, heart block, hypotension

Central nervous system

Irritability, headache

Gastrointestinal

Nausea

Respiratory

Dyspnea

Cautions/contraindications

♥ Do not use in second- or third-degree AV block.

♥ Adenosine is not effective in atrial flutter, atrial fibrillation, or ventricular tachycardia (arrhythmias **not due** to re-entry pathway through the AV or sinus node). In these cases, adenosine may be diagnostic, but not therapeutic.

Drug interactions

♥ If the patient is on caffeine or theophylline, higher doses may be required.

♥ If the patient is on digoxin or verapamil, lower doses may be required.

♥ If the patient is on carbamazepine, higher degrees of heart block may occur.

Patient monitoring

1. Notify the pediatric cardiologist, neonatologist, and health care providers of SVT.

2. Continue the rhythm strip through the "break" to normal sinus rhythm, or if SVT continues, for 1 minute.

3. If SVT stops, monitor the heart rate for conversion back to SVT.

4. If SVT continues, notify the pediatric cardiologist or neonatologist for further instructions.

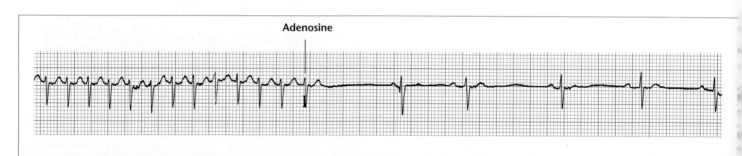

Figure 1.4. ECG of SVT treated with adenosine.

Vital Signs – Blood Pressure

Cuff size

For correct cuff size, measure the circumference of the upper arm. The width of the inflatable part of the cuff should be approximately 50% of the arm circumference. For example, if the arm circumference equals 15 cm, the width of the cuff should equal 7.5 cm.

* An undersized cuff overestimates the BP, giving false reassurance that the patient is normotensive, when in fact he is hypotensive.

* An oversized cuff underestimates the BP, showing that the patient is hypotensive, when in fact he is normotensive.

Methods for Measuring BP

Arterial

Common sites for arterial monitoring in neonates include the umbilical, radial, and posterior tibialis arteries. When the transducer is located at the level of the heart, the catheter and transducer are free of air bubbles, and the waveform is not dampened, arterial blood pressure is the most accurate method for assessing BP.

Oscillometric measurement

This is a non-invasive electronic method for measuring systolic, diastolic, and mean arterial blood pressure. Observe the same rules for cuff size presented above.

Ultrasonic doppler

This is a non-invasive method for measuring systolic blood pressure only. Apply the proper sized cuff to the arm or leg. Apply a conductive gel, and then interrogate the brachial (for arm BP) or posterior tibialis (for leg BP) pulse with the transducer. Inflate the cuff, then slowly deflate it. The systolic blood pressure will be the point on the manometer where the pulse becomes audible.

Normal

Blood pressure varies with age and weight.

When evaluating for congenital heart disease, a four-extremity blood pressure measurement may reveal discrepancies in blood pressure. In general, leg blood pressures are slightly higher than arm blood pressures, although they may be equal or slightly lower.

BP graphs are found in the blood pressure section of Part 3.

Abnormal

If the arm BP is more than 15 mmHg higher than the leg BP or the right arm BP is significantly higher than the left arm BP, consider coarctation of the aorta or interrupted aortic arch.

 Because hypotension is a late sign of cardiac decompensation, blood pressure may be normal when in fact the neonate is experiencing the early stages of shock. If the exam indicates the infant is underperfused, base the decision to treat on the physical exam, heart rate, and history, not on an isolated BP measurement!

Patient Assessment – Color (in well-lit room)

Normal

Pink skin color is normal. Assess mucous membranes in dark skinned neonates.

Acrocyanosis

Peripheral cyanosis or bluish discoloration of the hands and feet, not involving the mucous membranes, often resolves by 48 hours or with stabilization of the infant.

This results from an immature circulation or instability of the peripheral circulation, cold stress, shock, or polycythemia:

♥ Correct hypothermia if present.

♥ Evaluate for and treat shock.

♥ Measure the hemoglobin and hematocrit and treat polycythemia if indicated.

Circumoral cyanosis

Bluish discoloration around the mouth which is usually associated with nipple or breast feeding and should resolve following the feeding:

♥ Rule out central cyanosis.

Abnormal

Central cyanosis

Bluish discoloration of the tongue and mucous membranes caused by desaturation of arterial blood, indicates cardiac and/or respiratory dysfunction:

♥ Cyanosis may be visible with 3 to 5 gm/dL of reduced hemoglobin.

♥ Infants with polycythemia (Hgb > 20 gm) may appear cyanotic, even when adequately oxygenated.

♥ Infants with anemia (Hgb < 10 gm) may not appear cyanotic, even though severely hypoxemic.

Figure 1.5 displays the oxygen-hemoglobin dissociation curve and factors known to shift the curve to the left and right. An in-depth discussion of the O_2-hemoglobin dissociation curve may be found on page 116.

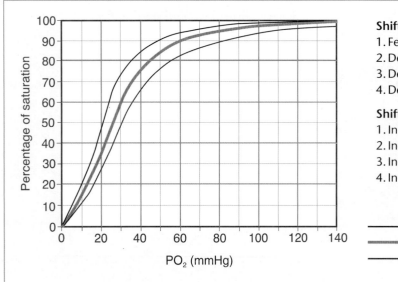

Shift-to-left curve:
1. Fetal hemoglobin
2. Decreased hydrogen ions (higher pH)
3. Decreased CO_2
4. Decreased temperature

Shift-to-right curve:
1. Increased hydrogen ions (lower pH)
2. Increased CO_2
3. Increased temperature
4. Increased 2,3-diphosphoglycerate (DPG)

——— Shift to left   pH 7.6
——— Normal   pH 7.4
——— Shift to right   pH 7.2

Figure 1.5. Oxygen-hemoglobin dissociation curve illustrating the curve lines for normal (center), left shift, and right shift.

Patient Assessment – Skin Perfusion (reflects cardiac output)

Normal

Capillary refill time is ≤ 3 seconds.

Abnormal

Signs of shock can be observed:

♥ Capillary refill time > 3 seconds

♥ Prolonged refill time in the lower body compared with the upper body

♥ Mottling, if associated with other symptoms

♥ Pallor

♥ Cool or cold extremities

♥ Cold sweat on the forehead/scalp (diaphoresis) caused by increased sympathetic activity as a response to decreased cardiac output

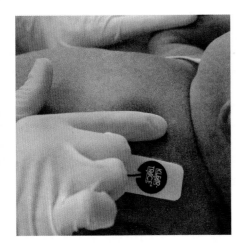 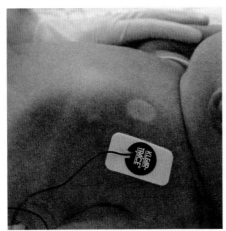 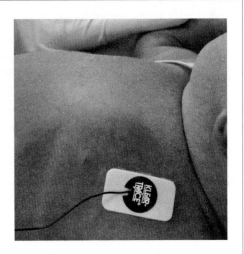

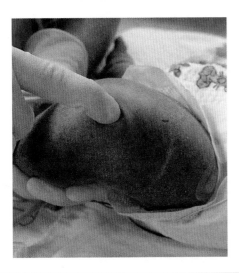 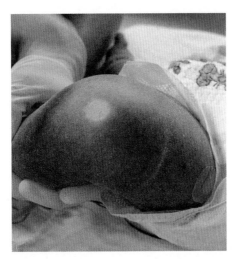

 Exam tip: Press firmly for five seconds to press the blood from the skin; then release and count how many seconds it takes for the skin to refill. Count "one-one thousand, two-one thousand . . ." until the skin refills with blood.

Figure 1.6. Procedure for checking capillary refill time in the upper and lower body. A comparison should be made between upper and lower capillary refill times.

Patient Assessment – Pulses (reflects cardiac output)

Normal

Pulses are usually easy to feel.

Brachial and femoral pulses are equal in strength.

Pedal pulses can be felt.

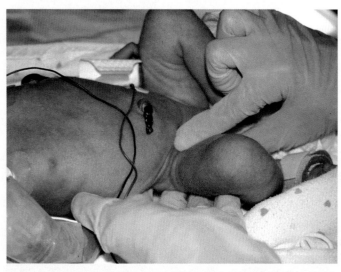

Figure 1.7. Palpating femoral pulses. Note the left hand under the hip to help raise the pelvis and open up the area for palpation.

 Exam tip: Palpate right, then left brachial artery; right, then left femoral artery; pedal arteries can be palpated separately or together. To improve skill level, perform this with every neonatal exam.

Abnormal

Discrepancy in pulse measurements may indicate an abnormality:

♥ Compare upper body to lower body.

♥ Compare right side to left side.

Pulses difficult to feel

Pulses that are difficult to palpate may indicate poor cardiac output and/or the presence of severe left heart obstructive lesions. When brachial pulses are palpable, but femoral pulses are weak or absent; or, when the right brachial pulse is stronger than the left brachial pulse, coarctation of the aorta or interrupted aortic arch should be considered.

Bounding pulses

Bounding pulses may be found in patent ductus arteriosus (PDA), aortic regurgitation, large arteriovenous malformation, truncus arteriosus.

Patient Assessment– Liver Size and Location

Normal

Located in the right abdomen, the liver edge should be ≤ 2 cm below the right costal margin.

Abnormal

Enlarged or misplaced liver

An enlarged liver, ≥ 3 cm below the right costal margin, is seen with congestive heart failure as the central venous pressure increases.

A midline location of the liver is seen with asplenia or polysplenia syndrome.

Liver located in the left abdomen

When the liver is in the left abdomen and the heart is in the right chest, this may represent *situs inversus totalis*, and the heart may be structurally normal (see figures 1.9 and 1.10).

When the liver is in the left abdomen and the heart is in the left chest, complex CHD is most likely present.

Bruits

If a bruit is auscultated over the liver or anterior fontanelle, consider evaluation for arteriovenous malformation (AVM).

A bruit heard over the carotid artery may indicate aortic stenosis (AS), especially if the murmur is loud at the upper right sternal border (URSB).

Some bruits over the carotid artery can be normal.

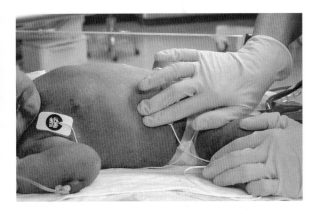

Figure 1.8. Examination of the liver must be performed when the infant is calm. Gently lifting and pressing the knees toward the chest may help to relax the abdominal muscles.

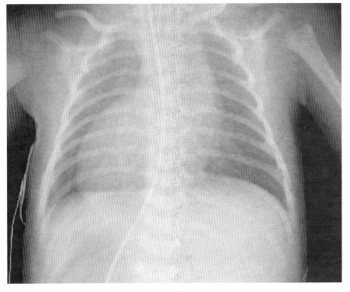

Figure 1.9. Chest x-ray of situs inversus totalis. Note the heart is in the right chest and the liver is in the left abdomen.

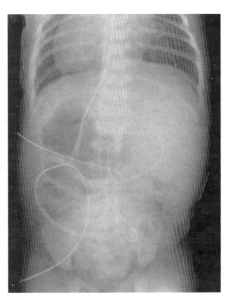

Figure 1.10. Abdominal x-ray of the same patient with situs inversus totalis. Note the gastric tube in the stomach, which is located in the right abdomen.

Patient Assessment – Neurologic Status

Normal

No signs of "distress" are observed.

The infant is active, alert, has good tone, a strong cry and a normal feeding pattern.

Abnormal

If the infant is in shock, he may display a range of symptoms including "distressed" facies, irritability, weak cry, lethargy, poor or flaccid tone, and if shock is advanced, a comatose state.

Early signs of deterioration include a poor feeding pattern, weak suck, and disinterest in feedings.

Patient Assessment – Infant Size and Appearance

Normal

The size of the infant's head, body length, and weight are all within normal limits or appropriate for gestational age (AGA).

The infant appears well-nourished.

Abnormal

Large for Gestational Age (LGA)

If the infant is large for gestational age (greater than the 90th percentile), evaluate for IDM and associated problems.

Infant of the diabetic mother (IDM)

Pre-existing and gestational diabetes is present in 1–4% of all pregnancies. Infants of diabetic mothers may have CHD, possibly due to interference with DNA-RNA transfer secondary to maternal high blood glucose before or at the time of conception and within the first 6 weeks of gestation. IDM patients suffer increased incidence of congenital heart defects, cardiomyopathy, and persistent pulmonary hypertension of the newborn (PPHN).

Hypertrophic cardiomyopathy

This occurs in 10–20% of IDM infants secondary to the effects of hyperinsulinemia, including increased myocardial fiber size and number. Hypertrophic cardiomyopathy can cause cardiomegaly and congestive heart failure. In some cases, left ventricular outflow tract obstruction occurs and results in a systolic ejection murmur. This condition usually resolves over the first few months of life, but may take as long as 12 months to resolve.

Congenital heart disease (CHD)

There is a 3–5% incidence of CHD in the IDM. This is 3 to 4 times greater than the incidence observed in the general population. The most common cardiac defects include:

- Transposition of the great arteries (TGA)
- Ventricular septal defect (VSD) and
- Coarctation of the aorta (COA)

Persistent pulmonary hypertension of the newborn (PPHN)

There is an increased incidence of PPHN secondary to concurrent conditions in the IDM that contribute to the persistence of pulmonary hypertension, including:

- Perinatal asphyxia
- Respiratory distress
- Polycythemia
- Hypoglycemia

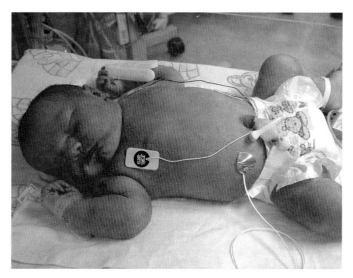

Figure 1.11. Large for gestational age, 36-week gestation infant of a diabetic mother.

Small for Gestational Age (SGA)

An infant is considered small for gestational age when body weight is less than the 10th percentile. Etiologies for growth restriction include maternal factors such as malnutrition, smoking, alcohol and drug use, hypertensive disorders, placental disease, advanced diabetes, and viral infection during pregnancy. Fetal factors that may be associated with growth restriction and SGA size include chromosomal (trisomy 21, 18, 13 and monosomy X) and genetic conditions.

Syndromes and Aneuploidy Associated with CHD

Neonates with chromosomal abnormalities are often SGA and have associated CHD.

Trisomy 21 (Down syndrome)

The incidence of Down syndrome is 1:650 births. Forty to 50 percent have cardiac defects; most common among them:

- ♥ Endocardial cushion defect (ECD)
- ♥ Ventricular septal defect (VSD)
- ♥ Atrial septal defect (ASD)
- ♥ Patent ductus arteriosus (PDA)
- ♥ Tetralogy of Fallot (TOF)

Physical features

Definitive physical features include small size, short round head with a flat facial profile, epicanthal folds, upslanting palpebral fissures, brushfield spots (speckling of the iris), small ears, short flat nasal bridge, protruding tongue, short narrow palate, open mouth, excess skin around the back of the neck, short fingers, square hands, clinodactyly (curving of the fifth finger inward), simian crease, wide gap between the first and second toes, poor moro reflex, hypotonia, hyperextensibility of the joints, broadened iliac bones, retarded psychomotor development, duodenal atresia, and umbilical hernia.

Trisomy 18 (Edwards syndrome)

The incidence of Edwards syndrome is 1:5000 to 1:7000 births; affected infants are three times more likely to be female than male. Ninety percent have cardiac defects; most common among them:

- ♥ Ventricular septal defect (VSD)
- ♥ Patent ductus arteriosus (PDA)
- ♥ Atrial septal defect (ASD)
- ♥ Pulmonic stenosis (PS)
- ♥ Polyvalvular disease

Physical features

Definitive physical features include small size (low birth weight), prominent occiput, narrowing of the bitemporal diameter, small palpebral fissures, ptosis of one or both eyelids, pinched appearance of the nose, low-set undeveloped ears, micrognathia, small mouth, short sternum, hands held in a clenched position with overlapping of the flexed third and fourth fingers by the second and fifth fingers (camptodactyly), hypoplastic nails, rocker bottom feet with protrusion of the calcaneus, umbilical hernia, and genitourinary defects.

Web sites for healthcare professionals and parents

www.marchofdimes.com National March of Dimes Web site

www.ndss.org National Down Syndrome Society Web site

www.trisomy.org A nonprofit volunteer organization offering support for parents who have had a child with a chromosome disorder, and education to families and professionals interested in the care of these children.

Patient Assessment – Infant Size and Appearance

Trisomy 13 (Patau syndrome)

The incidence of Patau syndrome is 1:7000 to 1:8000 births. Eighty to 90 percent have cardiac defects; most common among them:

♥ Ventricular septal defect (VSD)

♥ Patent ductus arteriosus (PDA)

♥ Atrial septal defect (ASD)

♥ Polyvalvular disease

♥ Dextrocardia

Physical features

Definitive physical features include small size (low birth weight), microcephaly, CNS malformations including holoprosencephaly, scalp defects, sloping forehead, central facial anomalies, midface hypoplasia-dysplasia, cleft lip and palate, coloboma of the iris, microphthalmia, anophthalmia, cataracts, hypotelorism, broad bulbous nose, low-set malformed ears, postaxial polydactyly, flexion deformities of the hands, fingers, and wrists, simian creases, rocker bottom feet, urogenital abnormalities, polycystic kidneys, omphalocele, inguinal or umbilical hernia, hypoplastic or absent ribs, and hypoplastic pelvis.

Monosomy X (Turner syndrome — XO)

The incidence of Turner syndrome is 1:2500 females. Only 5 percent of affected fetuses survive to term (95 percent are miscarried). Thirty-five percent have cardiac defects, including the following:

♥ Coarctation of the aorta (COA)

♥ Bicuspid aortic valve with variable stenosis

Physical features

Definitive physical features include short stature (mean birth weight 2900 grams), short webbed neck or redundant skin on the back of the neck, low posterior hairline, downslanted palpebral fissures, epicanthal folds and ptosis, micrognathia, low-set, posteriorly rotated ears, lymphedema of the dorsum of the hands and feet, broad thorax, widely spaced hypoplastic nipples, inguinal hernias, and hypoplastic convex nails.

Patient Assessment – Infant Size and Appearance

Dysmorphic Syndromes Associated with CHD

VATER association

Three or more associated defects are present:

Vertebral anomalies

Anal atresia

TracheoEsophageal fistula

Radial and Renal dysplasia

VACTERL association (expanded acronym)

Vertebral anomalies

Anal atresia

Cardiac defects

Tracheoesophageal fistula and/or Esophageal atresia

Renal agenesis and dysplasia

Limb anomalies (radial dysplasia—thumb or radial hypoplasia, polydactyly, syndactyly, radial club hand)

Variable incidence has been reported, ranging from 1:5500 births to 1.6:10,000 births. Fifty percent of affected individuals have cardiac defects, including:

♥ VSD

♥ TOF

♥ Double outlet right ventricle (DORV)

CHARGE association

Acronym stands for the following:

Coloboma

Heart defects

Atresia of the choanae

Retardation of growth and development

Genitourinary anomalies (genital hypoplasia)

Ear anomalies or deafness

Sixty-five to 85 percent of those affected have cardiac defects; most common among them:

♥ Aortic arch anomalies

♥ TOF

♥ Double outlet right ventricle (DORV)

♥ TOF with AV canal

♥ TOF with pulmonary atresia

♥ Truncus arteriosus

Patient Assessment – Infant Size and Appearance

22q11 deletion syndrome

This chromosome deletion is associated with most cases of DiGeorge, velocardiofacial, and conotruncal anomaly facial syndromes. The focus of this discussion is on DiGeorge syndrome, which is seen in 1 out of 32 neonates with congenital cardiac malformations. The most commonly associated lesions are the following:

♥ Interrupted aortic arch type B

♥ Truncus arteriosus

♥ TOF

♥ Pulmonary atresia with VSD

Physical features

Definitive physical features include downslanting eyes, hypertelorism, short philtrum, micrognathia, low-set posteriorly rotated ears, and "fish mouth" appearance.

Multisystem derangements

♥ Metabolic – including persistent hypocalcemia. Evaluate serum calcium and parathyroid hormone levels.

♥ Immunologic – including absent or hypoplastic thymus resulting in T-cell abnormalities. Evaluate a primary immunodeficiency panel. If transfusion is necessary, blood products should be irradiated to prevent graft-versus-host disease.

♥ Chromosomal – obtain a FISH chromosomal analysis for 22q11 deletion (definitive test).

Cardiac – Precordial Activity

Normal

Precordium
"Quiet" chest area immediately above the heart.

Point of maximal impulse (PMI)
In normal newborns, the PMI is located along the lower left sternal border in the fifth intercostal space.

Abnormal

Hyperactive precordium
If the PMI is in the right chest, consider:

- Dextrocardia (heart located in the right chest)
- Left-sided diaphragmatic hernia
- Tension left pneumothorax

If the PMI is in the left axilla, consider:

- Right pneumothorax

Thrill
A vibratory sensation associated with a loud harsh murmur is known as a thrill. The location of a thrill depends on the defect:

- Upper left sternal border (ULSB) – pulmonary artery or valve origin, e.g., pulmonary stenosis
- Upper right sternal border (URSB) – aortic origin, e.g., aortic stenosis
- Lower left sternal border (LLSB) – ventricular septal defect (VSD)
- Suprasternal notch – aortic stenosis

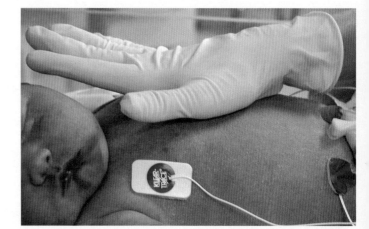

Figure 1.12. Palpating the chest to evaluate the precordium for a thrill. The outstretched palm of the hand should be gently moved over the chest to detect a thrill in the ULSB, URSB, or LLSB.

 Exam tip: Palpate the chest lightly with the palm of your hand. To improve skill level, perform this with every neonatal exam.

Cardiac – Heart Sounds

First heart sound – S1

Associated with closure of the mitral and tricuspid valves at the end of atrial systole, S1 is heard best at the fifth intercostal space at the left midclavicular line or LLSB.

Second heart sound – S2

Associated with closure of the aortic and pulmonic valves at the end of ventricular systole, S2 is heard best at the ULSB.

Splitting of S1

This may be normal, but is infrequently heard.

Splitting of S2

Two components of the second heart sound are audible with inspiration; closure of the aortic (A2), then pulmonic (P2) valves: S2 = A2, P2. S2 becomes a single sound with expiration.

A single S2 is normal in the first several days of life because of increased pulmonary vascular resistance.

It is difficult to hear splitting of S2 with tachycardia.

Exam tip: Normally a physical exam is conducted from head to toe. When listening to heart sounds, work in the opposite order: Start low and move up. Listen carefully, then move the stethoscope from the LLSB fifth intercostal space straight up to the ULSB area. The first heart sound will be louder in the low position and the second heart sound will be louder in the higher position.

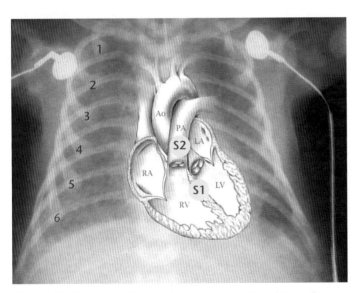

Figure 1.13. Illustration of the heart showing where S1 and S2 are best heard. The anterior ribs are numbered over the right chest. S1 is best heard at the apex at the fifth intercostal space. S2 is best heard over the ULSB.

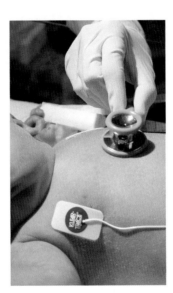
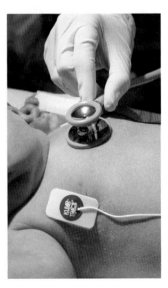

Figure 1.14. Ausculation of heart sounds. Note that the stethoscope is placed over the area where S1 is loudest, then moved up to the area where S2 is loudest.

Cardiac – Heart Sounds

Abnormal

Widely split S1

A widely split S1 is associated with the following:

♥ Bundle branch block

♥ Ebstein's anomaly

Widely split S2

A widely split S2 may indicate the following:

♥ Right bundle branch block

♥ Early aortic closure

♥ Atrial septal defect (ASD)

♥ Total anomalous pulmonary venous return (TAPVR), without obstruction

♥ Pulmonary stenosis (PS)

♥ Ebstein's anomaly

Narrowly split S2

A narrowly split S2 is associated with the following:

♥ Aortic stenosis (AS)

♥ Pulmonary hypertension

♥ May be a normal finding

Single S2

A single S2 represents absence of either the aortic (A2) or pulmonic (P2) valve component as in the following conditions:

♥ Severe aortic stenosis (AS)

♥ Aortic atresia (AA)

♥ Severe pulmonary stenosis (PS)

♥ Pulmonary atresia (PAtr)

♥ Truncus arteriosus (Truncus)

♥ Pulmonary hypertension

♥ Transposition of the Great Arteries (TGA)

♥ Tetralogy of Fallot (TOF)

Cardiac – Heart Murmur

What is a heart murmur?

Sound caused by turbulent blood flow, due to one of the following conditions:

♥ Blood forced through narrowed passageways, as in valvular stenosis and ventricular septal defect

♥ Regurgitation through incompetent or abnormal valves

♥ Increased blood flow across normal structures, as in anemia

Loudness/intensity

Grade 1   Barely audible

Grade 2   Soft but audible

Grade 3   Moderately loud, no thrill

Grade 4   Loud and associated with a thrill

Grade 5   Audible with a stethoscope barely on the chest

Grade 6   Audible with the stethoscope not touching the chest

Timing

Systolic

Heard between the first and second heart sound — S1 and S2

Diastolic

Heard between the second and first heart sound — S2 and S1

Continuous

Heard throughout systole and extending into diastole

Quality descriptors

♥ Musical

♥ Vibratory (high or low-pitched)

♥ Harsh

♥ Blowing

> ⚠ *An infant with NO heart murmur may still have significant cardiac disease.*

Exam tip: When listening for a heart murmur, it does not matter in which order you move the stethoscope on the chest. The most important thing is to be systematic in your approach. One method to consider: listen carefully at the upper right sternal border (URSB), then the upper left sternal border (ULSB), then slide the stethoscope down to the lower right sternal border (LRSB), then to the apex. Auscultate the axillae and posterior lung fields. A systematic approach will help determine the following characteristics of a murmur:

♦ *Timing*

♦ *Location*

♦ *Loudness/intensity*

♦ *Quality*

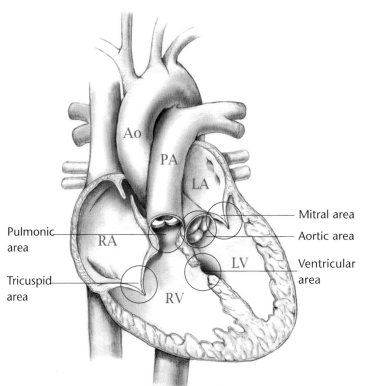

Figure 1.15. Illustration of the heart showing locations where cardiac murmurs may originate.

Cardiac – Heart Murmur

Normal

Non-pathologic murmurs

Peripheral pulmonic stenosis (PPS)

♥ Short systolic ejection murmur

♥ Grade 1-2/6

♥ Heard loudest in the axillae and back (posterior lung fields); also heard at the upper left sternal border (ULSB)

Systolic ejection or continuous murmur

♥ Grade 1-2/6

♥ Often heard in the first week of life as pulmonary vascular resistance decreases and the ductus arteriosus closes

Abnormal

Pathologic murmurs

Murmurs are usually pathologic if associated with any of the following:

Signs and symptoms

♥ Central cyanosis

♥ Respiratory distress

♥ Abnormal pulses, perfusion

♥ Shock

Abnormal physical exam

♥ ≥ Grade 3 murmur within hours of birth

♥ Gallop

♥ A pansystolic murmur can be heard with CHD (regurgitant systolic murmur secondary to mitral or tricuspid regurgitation), with severe pulmonary disease (tricuspid regurgitation), or with injury to the tricuspid valve secondary to asphyxia.

♥ A diastolic murmur is always abnormal and is usually associated with abnormalities of the aortic or pulmonic valves (aortic or pulmonic valve regurgitation).

♥ A continuous murmur is a associated with patent ductus arteriosus (PDA) or arteriovenous malformation (AVM) located in the brain or liver; and is especially concerning if associated with signs of congestive heart failure.

Abnormal chest x-ray

♥ Abnormal size or shape of the heart

♥ Increased or decreased pulmonary vascularity

Neonates with congenital heart disease usually present with one or more of the following signs or symptoms:

- Central cyanosis

- Heart murmur

- Tachypnea

- Respiratory distress

- Congestive heart failure

- Signs of poor cardiac output (poor pulses, mottling, hypotension, metabolic acidosis, circulatory compromise)

- Abnormal heart rhythm (tachycardia, bradycardia, heart block)

- Abnormal heart size, shape, location

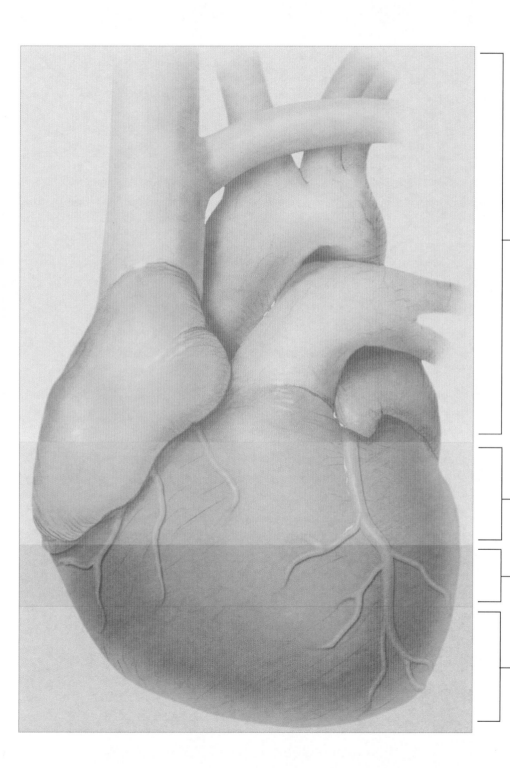

All other congenital heart
defects — 58%

Cyanotic CHD, not ductal
dependent — 15%

Cyanotic CHD, ductal dependent
for pulmonary blood flow — 9%

Left outflow tract CHD, ductal
dependent for systemic blood
flow — 18%

History and General Presentation

When a neonate presents with cyanosis, respiratory distress, and/or shock, the process of determining whether signs and symptoms are due to pulmonary, cardiac, infectious, neurologic, or other causes begins. Information valuable to differential diagnosis includes the following:

Family, pregnancy, and maternal medical history

a) A sibling with congenital heart disease (CHD) increases the recurrence risk for CHD three-fold. When several siblings are affected, the risk for CHD increases substantially to 10%. If the mother has CHD, the risk of CHD in her offspring is increased.

b) Maternal ingestion, early in pregnancy, of alcohol, recreational drugs, and both prescription and over-the-counter medications, increases the risk for heart defects, as does viral exposure during pregnancy (see Table 2.1).

c) Pregnancy, labor, and delivery complications should be carefully evaluated for risk factors that could affect the cardiovascular system or conditions that mimic CHD. For example, intrauterine or perinatal hypoxia are risk factors for the development of myocardial dysfunction, as well as persistent pulmonary hypertension of the newborn (PPHN). Risk factors for sepsis should be identified, as septic neonates may present in shock similarly to those with left heart obstructive lesions. Other causes of shock, including maternal/fetal hemorrhage, should be identified and treated.

Table 2.1. Congenital Heart Defects Associated with Maternal Alcohol or Drug Use and Infections

Drugs	
Alcohol	VSD, ASD, TOF
Amphetamines	VSD, PDA, ASD, TGA
Anticonvulsants	
Dilantin	PS, AS, COA, VSD
Trimethadione	TGA, TOF, HLHS
Lithium	Ebstein's anomaly
Hormones Progesterone, estrogen	VSD, TGA, TOF
Viral Infection	
Rubella	PDA, branch PA stenosis, VSD, ASD, myocarditis, hydrops
Coxsackie B virus and enteroviruses	Viral myocarditis, pericarditis
Medical Conditions	
Diabetes	TGA, VSD, COA, hypertrophic cardiomyopathy
Systemic lupus erythematosus and connective tissue disorders	Complete heart block and cardiomyopathy
Maternal age > 40	TOF, Trisomy 21 with risk of associated CHD

VSD (ventricular septal defect), ASD (atrial septal defect), TOF (tetralogy of Fallot), PDA (patent ductus arteriosus), TGA (transposition of the great arteries), PS (pulmonary stenosis), AS (aortic stenosis), COA (coarctation of the aorta), HLHS (hypoplastic left heart syndrome), PA (pulmonary artery)

History and General Presentation

Neonatal history, including gestational age, symptoms at onset, and severity of symptoms

Within the first week of life, a baby who presents with severe cyanosis, congestive heart failure, and/or cardiovascular collapse must be evaluated for congenital heart disease. The timing and history of symptom onset is very important. A term infant who has been well the first few days of life, but who becomes tachypneic, feeds poorly, and displays signs of shock should prompt consideration of left outflow tract obstruction with a closing ductus arteriosus. The infant with early onset respiratory distress following a difficult birth, or born to a group B streptococcus positive mother, is more likely suffering from pulmonary disease or the effects of sepsis. A premature infant is more likely to have pulmonary causes of respiratory distress, although cardiac disease does occur in both prematurely born and term infants. In general, the cyanotic infant without significant respiratory distress must be evaluated for cardiac disease; such a presentation is not uncommon with cyanotic congenital heart disease.

A complete physical examination and evaluation of vital signs

Details are given in Part 1.

Chest x-ray

a) Determine whether pulmonary vascular markings are decreased, normal, or increased. An increased heart size with increased pulmonary vascular markings or pulmonary edema may indicate heart defects with increased pulmonary blood flow or left outflow tract obstruction (see Figure 2.1). An enlarged heart size may also be seen following asphyxial injury to the myocardium or heart valves. A normal or small-sized heart associated with decreased pulmonary vascular markings may be seen with heart lesions with decreased pulmonary blood flow (see figures 2.2 and 2.3). Pulmonary vascular markings may also be decreased with persistent pulmonary hypertension of the newborn (PPHN).

b) The presence of infiltrates, pleural effusions, air leaks, or chest masses, especially when associated with a normal heart size, correlates more often with respiratory causes or sepsis (see Figure 2.4). Pulmonary edema is often associated with lesions characterized by obstruction to pulmonary venous drainage or left heart obstruction and congestive heart failure.

c) The degree of lung inflation may also help distinguish between pulmonary and cardiac disease. Atelectasis with air bronchograms is present in respiratory distress syndrome (RDS). Atelectasis without air bronchograms may be seen with hypoventilation secondary to neurologic or respiratory depression. Overinflation can occur when an infant with cardiac disease, but normal lung compliance, is ventilated. Pneumonia and total anomalous pulmonary venous return (TAPVR) should be considered when a neonate presents with marked respiratory distress and radiographic appearance of a reticulogranular pattern, lack of air bronchograms, and overinflation of the lungs.

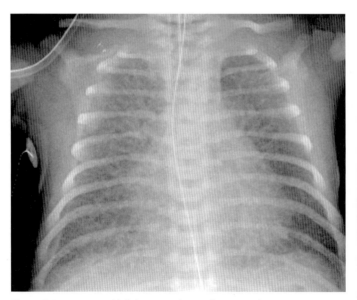

Figure 2.1. Neonate with left ventricular outflow tract obstruction. Cardiomegaly and congestive failure are evident. Note the interstitial and alveolar edema and small bilateral pleural effusions, right greater than left.

History and General Presentation

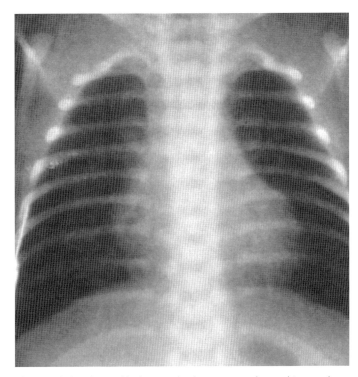

Figure. 2.2. Newborn with decreased pulmonary vascular markings and a normal heart size.

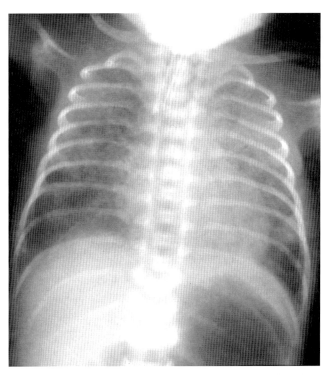

Figure 2.4. Newborn with pulmonary hemorrhage. Note the asymmetric pattern of infiltrates with the left side more affected than the right.

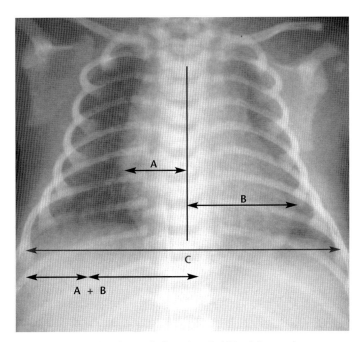

Figure 2.3. Measuring the cardiothoracic ratio (CT ratio) to evaluate heart size.

Table 2.2. Measuring the CT Ratio to Estimate Heart Size

1. Measure A + B.

 A = widest horizontal diameter right of midline.

 B = widest horizontal diameter left of midline.

2. Measure C.

 C = widest internal diameter of the chest at, or just below the base of the heart.

3. A + B divided by C equals the CT ratio.

 CT ratio < 60% in the neonate is considered normal (A + B < 60% of C).

A CT ratio > 60% is considered enlarged.

 Ascertain the x-ray being evaluated reflects a good inspiration and that the infant is not rotated.

Both inadequate inspiration and rotation may make the heart appear enlarged.

Oximetry

a) Infants presenting with cyanosis are provided oxygen to improve arterial oxygenation. Cyanotic CHD should be suspected when there is a minimal increase in O_2 saturation or arterial PO_2 when the infant breathes 100% oxygen. A hyperoxia (oxygen-challenge) test is useful to evaluate the arterial PO_2 when the infant breathes 100% oxygen. However, this test is not 100% sensitive for CHD, (see Part 3 for details on performing this test.) Infants presenting with shock may suffer from left heart obstruction. The saturation and PaO_2 is usually responsive to oxygen administration, yet the cardiac defect is severe.

b) Differences in pre-and post-ductal saturation should be noted (see Part 3 for details). A higher saturation in the right hand compared to the foot indicates a right-to-left ductal shunt. *Reverse differential cyanosis*, a lower saturation in the right hand compared to the foot, suggests transposition of the great arteries.

Respiratory versus metabolic acidosis

CO_2 retention with respiratory acidosis is more likely to be observed with lung disease caused by pneumonia, respiratory distress syndrome, aspiration, or other pulmonary diseases. Hypoxemia and/or shock often accompany serious heart disease, with tachypnea the normal compensatory result. When lung compliance is normal as is often the case in CHD, the tachypneic infant readily exhales CO_2, which leads to hypocarbia. Therefore, metabolic acidosis with a normal or low CO_2 is more often observed with CHD, although a mixed pattern of metabolic and respiratory acidosis is possible. Neonates with bacterial sepsis also commonly present with hypoxemia and metabolic and/or respiratory acidosis; therefore sepsis must be included in the differential diagnosis.

History and General Presentation

Diagnostic tests

a) An electrocardiogram (ECG) is an essential test for evaluating and managing arrhythmias. If consultation is desired, an ECG can be faxed to a pediatric cardiologist. Although some ECG changes may suggest specific abnormalities (left axis deviation with endocardial cushion defects or tricuspid atresia), more often, the ECG changes are nonspecific.

b) An echocardiogram is the most definitive test to confirm congenital heart disease and should be performed whenever congenital heart disease is suspected.

Table 2.3. Chest X-ray Evaluation

The following items should be assessed:

- Quality — rotation, penetration, inflation
- Heart size — small, normal, enlarged
- Heart shape and location
- Pulmonary vascular markings — decreased vs. increased

- Presence of pulmonary edema
- Infiltrates — symmetric vs. asymmetric
- Mediastinum — narrow, normal, wide

- Air leaks — pneumothorax, pneumomediastinum

- Central line location
- Tube location — endotracheal, gastric, chest

Table 2.4. Pulmonary versus Cardiac Disease

	Pulmonary	Cardiac
Cyanosis	Yes	Yes
Respiratory rate	Increased	Increased – often described as "comfortably tachypneic"
Work of breathing	Increased	Easy effort; but increased if CHF has developed
Acid/base balance	Increased PCO_2 Respiratory acidosis more common	Decreased PCO_2 Metabolic acidosis more common unless there is concurrent pulmonary disease
Chest X-ray	Asymmetric pattern of infiltrates or other pulmonary disease	Increased or decreased pulmonary vascular markings; pulmonary edema*
Heart size, shape, location	Normal	Abnormal
O_2 challenge test	PO_2 >150	PO_2 <150 (cyanotic CHD)

*May have infiltrates or other findings consistent with concurrent pulmonary disease

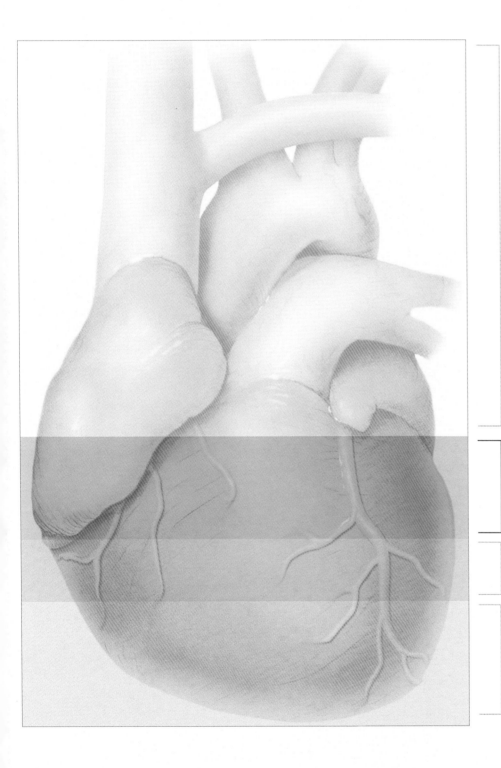

Cyanotic CHD
Not ductal dependent

All other congenital heart defects — 58%

Tetralogy of Fallot* — 10%

Truncus arteriosus — 1–3%

Total anomalous pulmonary venous return — 1%

Ebstein's anomaly* — <1%

Cyanotic CHD, ductal dependent for pulmonary blood flow — 9%

Left outflow tract CHD, ductal dependent for systemic blood flow — 18%

*Extreme forms may be ductal dependent

General approach recommended for cyanotic neonates with suspected CHD

1. Provide 100% oxygen and other respiratory support as indicated.

2. Evaluate for physical and laboratory signs of shock and offer resuscitative care as indicated.

3. Carefully evaluate the neonate for any other causes of cyanosis as previously discussed (e.g. pulmonary disease, sepsis, shock secondary to non-cardiac causes, and neurologic depression).

4. Following this evaluation, if cardiac disease is suspected, the O_2 saturation remains less than 75%, and an echocardiogram is not readily available, then a Prostaglandin E_1 infusion should be considered. Since this medication may cause serious side effects including hypotension and apnea, (see page 66), its use should be carefully evaluated.

 Infants with suspected left heart obstructive lesions (coarctation of the aorta, interrupted aortic arch, hypoplastic left heart, and critical aortic stenosis) may present in shock without severe cyanosis.

Underlying Concepts

- Neonates with cyanotic congenital heart disease (CHD) have mixing of red (oxygenated, saturated) and blue (deoxygenated, desaturated) blood at the atrial and/or ventricular level.

- Blood must flow through the pulmonary artery to the lungs to become oxygenated.

- When blood is diverted away from the pulmonary artery and lungs by a right-to-left shunt at the atrial and/or ventricular level, a higher volume of blue blood will be ejected through the aorta — to the body — and the infant will appear cyanotic.

- Cyanosis improves with improved pulmonary blood flow. As a larger volume of blue blood enters the lungs, a larger volume of oxygenated red blood will return via the pulmonary veins to the heart. Thus the proportion of red to blue blood will increase and cyanosis will decrease or disappear.

- Unless the neonate has one of the most severe forms of tetralogy or Ebstein's anomaly, adequate amounts of blood will circulate to the lungs and body without the help of a patent ductus arteriosus.

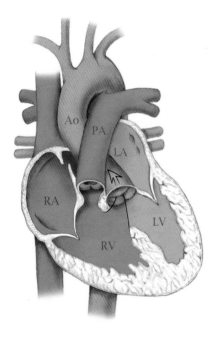

Tetralogy of Fallot

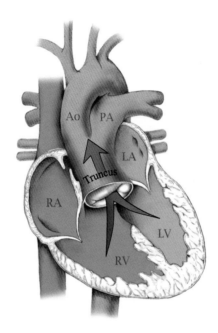

Truncus arteriosus

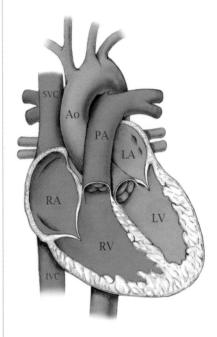

Normal heart

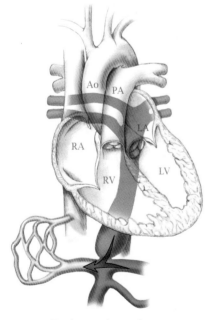

Total anomalous pulmonary
venous return

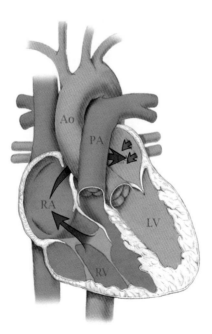

Ebstein's anomaly

Figure 2.5. Comparative illustrations of the CHD lesions that are not ductal dependent.

Tetralogy of Fallot (TOF)

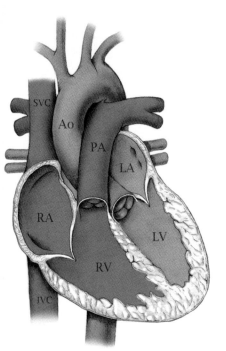

Normal heart

TOF affects approximately 10% of all infants with congenital heart disease. Four main abnormalities characterize the disorder: a large ventricular septal defect (VSD), right ventricular hypertrophy, right ventricular outflow tract obstruction, and aortic override of the ventricular septum. Severity of symptoms relates to the degree of right ventricular outflow tract obstruction (degree of pulmonary stenosis or the presence of pulmonary atresia).

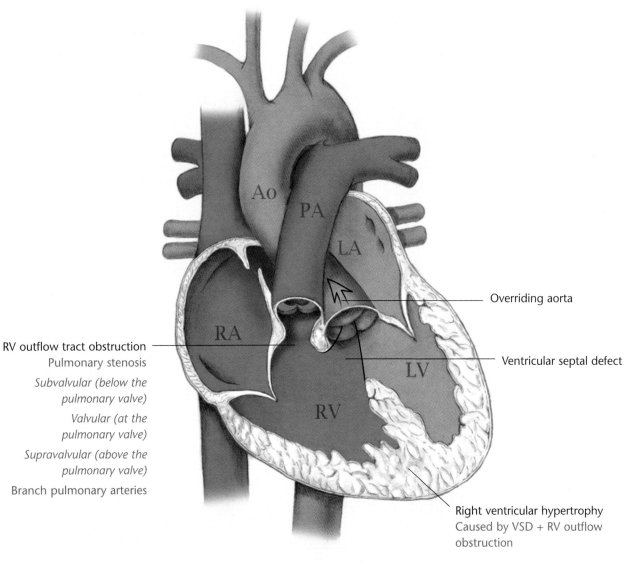

RV outflow tract obstruction
Pulmonary stenosis
Subvalvular (below the pulmonary valve)
Valvular (at the pulmonary valve)
Supravalvular (above the pulmonary valve)
Branch pulmonary arteries

Overriding aorta

Ventricular septal defect

Right ventricular hypertrophy
Caused by VSD + RV outflow obstruction

Figure 2.6. Anatomic features of TOF.

39

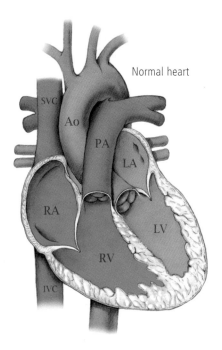

Normal heart

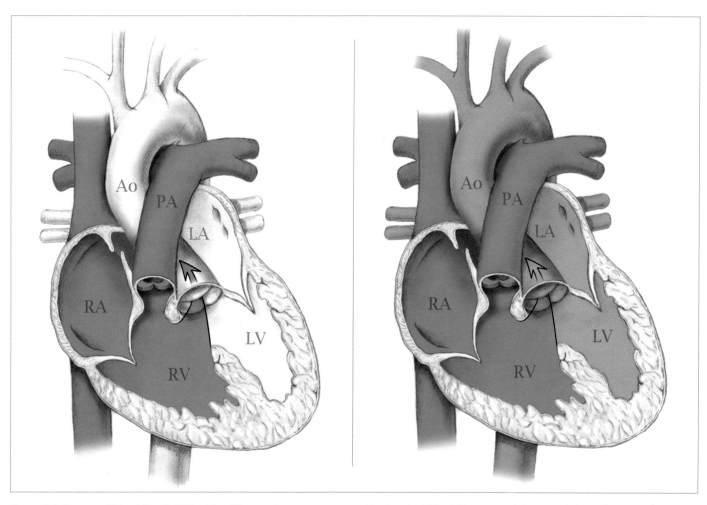

Figure 2.7. Pattern of blood flow in TOF with mild to moderate pulmonary stenosis (PS). Note the right-to-left shunting of deoxygenated blood at the VSD, which may result in cyanosis depending upon the amount of deoxygenated blood entering the aorta.

Tetralogy of Fallot (TOF)

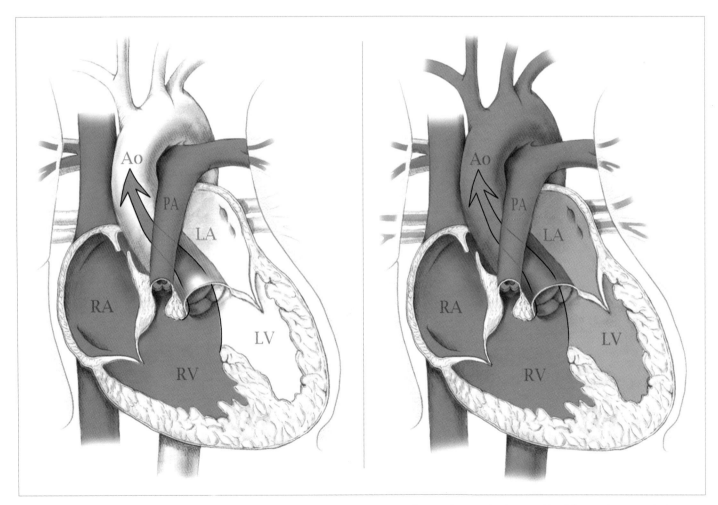

Figure 2.8. TOF with more severe PS. The right outflow tract obstruction causes an increased amount of blood to shunt right-to-left through the VSD. Notice the lower volume of blood in the pulmonary arteries and veins, reflecting decreased pulmonary blood flow and return. A higher proportion of blue to red blood entering the systemic circulation will result in the appearance of cyanosis.

Tetralogy of Fallot (TOF)

Clinical Presentation

Severity of cyanosis varies depending upon the degree of right ventricular outflow tract obstruction.

When pulmonary stenosis is mild, blood flow to the lungs is not restricted. In addition to normal blood flow through the pulmonary artery, blood also shunts from the left ventricle through the VSD to the pulmonary artery and lungs. This is called a left-to-right shunt and results in excessive pulmonary blood flow. This type of tetralogy is called acyanotic tetralogy or a "pink tet."

With more pronounced pulmonary stenosis, blood flow to the lungs is restricted: blue (deoxygenated) blood shunts from the right ventricle through the VSD and out the aorta. This is called a right-to-left shunt. A smaller amount of blood enters the lungs, therefore, a smaller amount also returns from the lungs. The proportion of "blue" blood to "red" blood entering the aorta is higher and cyanosis may become apparent. If pulmonary stenosis is significant or pulmonary atresia is present, a prostaglandin E_1 infusion is necessary to open and maintain ductal patency.

Murmur

Caused by the pulmonary stenosis (not the VSD) and audible at birth.

With worsening pulmonary stenosis, the murmur can become shorter and softer.

Increased intensity of the murmur → decreased pulmonary stenosis.
Decreased intensity of the murmur → increased pulmonary stenosis.

Single S2

The pulmonary component (P2) of the second heart sound is not audible.

Chest X-ray

Heart size
Heart size is usually normal.

Heart shape
The concave main PA segment with upturned apex, secondary to right ventricular hypertrophy, creates the appearance of a "boot shaped" heart.

Variable pulmonary vascular markings
Pulmonary vascular markings will decrease (the lung fields will appear dark) when there is decreased pulmonary blood flow, as seen with severe pulmonary stenosis or pulmonary atresia. In contrast, when the pulmonary stenosis is mild, pulmonary vascularity may be increased.

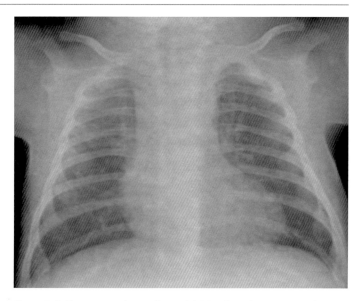

Figure 2.9 Chest x-ray of a newborn with TOF. The pulmonary vascular markings are not decreased, reflecting adequate pulmonary blood flow. A normal-sized "boot-shaped" heart is apparent.

Tetralogy of Fallot (TOF)

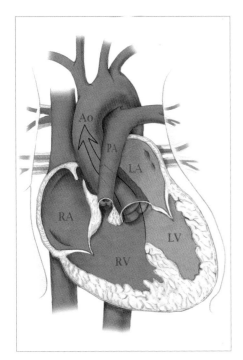

TOF with restricted pulmonary blood flow.

Initial Stabilization

1. Provide supplemental oxygen to treat cyanosis and help relax the pulmonary vascular bed. The majority of infants with tetralogy are not ductal dependent.

2. If the O_2 saturation remains < 75% on oxygen, the infant may have significant pulmonary stenosis or atresia. Until the diagnosis can be confirmed by echocardiogram, begin a prostaglandin E_1 infusion to maintain ductal patency. See page 66 for details about prostaglandin infusions.

3. If the O_2 saturation is > 75%, cardiology consultation should be requested to allow further evaluation.

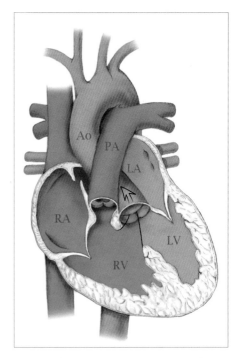

TOF with adequate pulmonary blood flow.

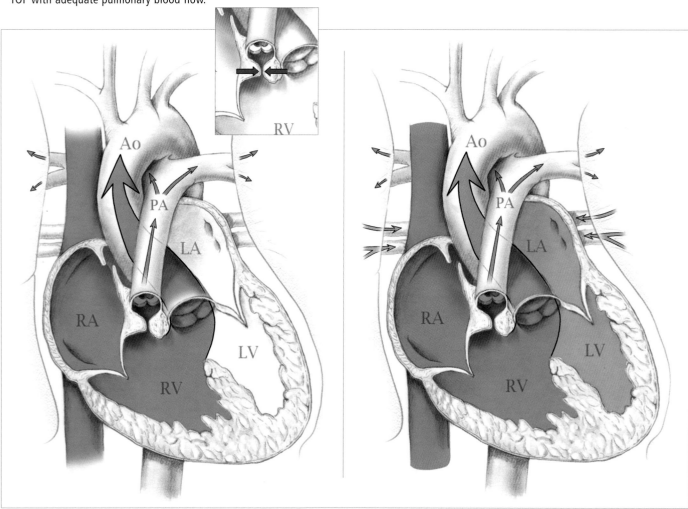

Figure 2.10. Pattern of blood flow seen during a "tet" spell. Severe right outflow tract obstruction causes most of the blood entering the right ventricle to shunt right-to-left through the VSD. Pulmonary blood flow is markedly reduced, resulting in severe hypoxemia and cyanosis.

Tet (Hypoxic) Spell

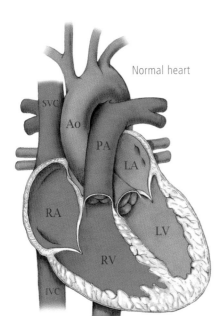
Normal heart

Also called a cyanotic or hypercyanotic spell, infants experiencing a tet spell become irritable, progressively hypoxemic, pale, hyperpneic (increased rate and depth of respirations), flaccid, and at times, suffer loss of consciousness. Severe hypoxemia during a tet spell may severely impact the central nervous and other organ systems. Immediate recognition and treatment is therefore imperative.

Hypoxemia ➔ stimulates the respiratory center ➔ rapid, deep respirations (hyperpnea) ➔ negative thoracic pump becomes more efficient ➔ increases systemic venous return ➔ increases right-to-left shunting.

What causes a tet spell?

During a tet spell, blood flow across the right ventricular outflow tract is significantly decreased, resulting in shunting right-to-left through the VSD and out the aorta, thus bypassing the lungs. Various theories have been offered to account for the cause of tet spells, including "spasm" of the right ventricular outflow tract (shown on page 44), and/or a sudden decrease in systemic vascular resistance secondary to hypovolemia, dehydration, hot weather, or defecation. *Tet spells are usually not seen in the neonatal period, and peak in incidence between 2 and 4 months of life.*

Blood flow during a tet spell.

Principles of Treatment

1. Calm the infant.

2. Increase systemic vascular resistance to decrease the right-to-left shunt at the VSD.

3. Improve pulmonary blood flow and ultimately improve arterial oxygenation and saturation.

Inpatient care

Calm the infant

To decrease oxygen demands and relieve anxiety, attempt to calm the crying irritable infant by non-pharmacologic methods initially. When usual calming techniques fail, morphine or other sedatives may be necessary.

Increase systemic vascular resistance to decrease the right-to-left shunt at the VSD

♥ Place the infant in a knee-chest position. If the infant can tolerate being lifted, place the baby over your shoulder with the knees drawn up toward the chest. If lifting is not possible, press the knees up toward the chest (if lying supine), or lay the infant prone and tuck the knees up against the chest. This position will increase peripheral resistance in the lower extremities and increase systemic vascular resistance. This will decrease the right-to-left shunt through the VSD and improve pulmonary blood flow.

♥ Infusion of volume expanders may also be helpful to increase systemic vascular resistance.

♥ Peripheral vasoconstrictors such as phenylephrine may be necessary to increase systemic vascular resistance, help reduce the shunt at the VSD, and therefore promote pulmonary blood flow.

Tet (Hypoxic) Spell

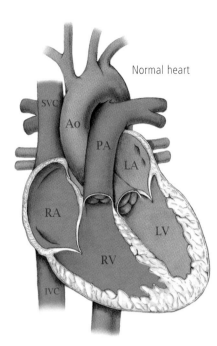

Normal heart

Improve pulmonary blood flow and ultimately improve arterial oxygenation and saturation

- Administer oxygen to help improve arterial saturation, understanding there may be little to no improvement until pulmonary blood flow increases.

- Hyperpnea, or an increased rate and depth of respirations, often accompanies the onset of a tet spell. During hyperpnea, the negative thoracic pump becomes more efficient and increases systemic venous return to the right heart. This in turn, increases the right-to-left shunt at the VSD. Attempt to abolish hyperpnea by using morphine or other sedative medications. If intravenous access is not available, morphine may be given by the intramuscular route.

- During prolonged and/or severe spells, support of ventilation may be necessary.

- Hypoxemia during a tet spell may lead to the development of metabolic acidosis. Relieve tissue hypoxia (improve oxygenation and perfusion) as rapidly as possible to reverse acidosis and reduce its negative impact on the respiratory center and pulmonary vasculature.

- In severe cases, sodium bicarbonate may be necessary to help correct acidosis. Do not administer this medication if the patient is not adequately ventilated.

Outpatient treatment, parental education

1. Calm the baby.

2. Instruct the parents to hold the infant over their shoulder with his knees drawn up toward his chest.

3. Instruct the parents to contact a pediatric cardiologist if the infant is not improving, or take the baby to the emergency room.

47

Type 1

The main pulmonary artery arises from the truncal root and bifurcates into the right and left pulmonary arteries.

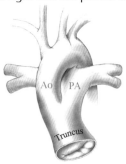

Type 2

Separate origins of the right and left pulmonary artery arise from the posterior truncal root.

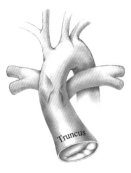

Type 3

Same as Type 2 except the pulmonary arteries arise from the lateral sides of the truncal root.

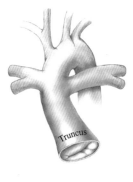

Figure 2.11. The three main types of truncus arteriosus.

Truncus Arteriosus

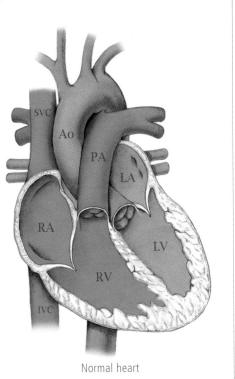

Normal heart

Truncus arteriosus affects approximately 1–3% of all neonates with CHD. Three main subtypes are based on the origin of the pulmonary arteries. Type 1 and Type 2 account for 85% of truncus arteriosus cases. Other findings include a 33% incidence of 22q11 deletion syndrome, 30% incidence of right aortic arch, and 10–20% incidence of interrupted aortic arch. If interrupted aortic arch is present, systemic blood flow is dependent upon the ductus arteriosus, and a prostaglandin E_1 infusion will be necessary to maintain ductal patency.

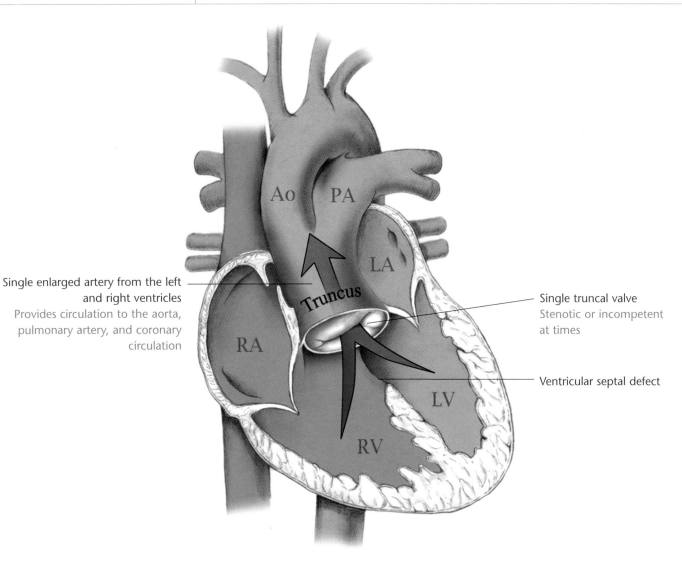

Single enlarged artery from the left and right ventricles
Provides circulation to the aorta, pulmonary artery, and coronary circulation

Single truncal valve
Stenotic or incompetent at times

Ventricular septal defect

Figure 2.12 Anatomic features of truncus arteriosus Type 1.

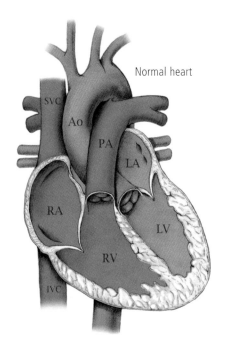

Normal heart

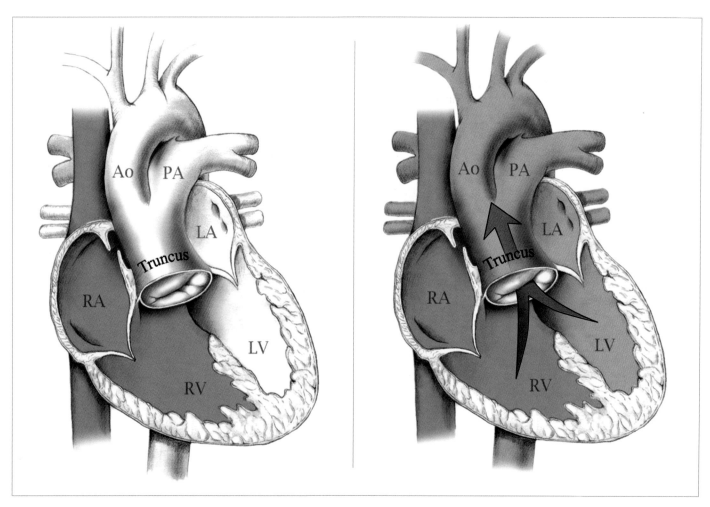

Figure 2.13. Blood flow pattern in truncus arteriosus. Deoxygenated blood from the right ventricle mixes with oxygenated blood from the left ventricle at the VSD and is ejected through the truncal root to the systemic, pulmonary, and coronary circulation.

Truncus Arteriosus

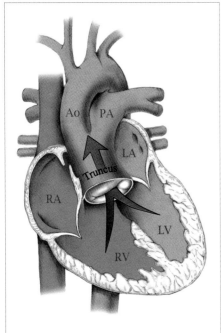

Truncus arteriosus Type 1

Clinical Presentation

Cyanosis
Mixing of oxygenated with deoxygenated blood leads to arterial desaturation and sometimes cyanosis.

Congestive heart failure (CHF)
As pulmonary vascular resistance (PVR) decreases in the neonatal period, blood flow to the lungs increases and leads to pulmonary overcirculation and CHF. Signs and symptoms of CHF, which may develop several days to several weeks after birth, include tachypnea, bounding pulses, tiring and dyspnea (shortness of breath) with feeds, and diaphoresis.

↑ PVR → decreased pulmonary blood flow → increased cyanosis.

↓ PVR → increased pulmonary blood flow → decreased or no cyanosis.

Heart sounds
Distinguishing heart sounds include a loud single S2 and a loud ejection click.

Murmur
A systolic ejection murmur may be heard at the ULSB or URSB. A diastolic murmur may be heard if the truncal valve is regurgitant.

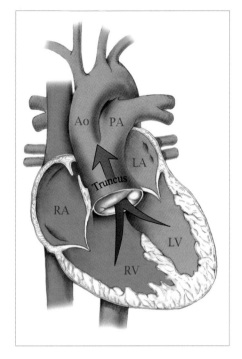

Truncus arteriosus Type 1

Chest X-ray

Heart size
Moderate cardiomegaly is usually apparent.

Pulmonary Vascular Markings
Increased pulmonary vascular markings are apparent secondary to increased pulmonary blood flow.

Other
30 percent occurrence of a right aortic arch.

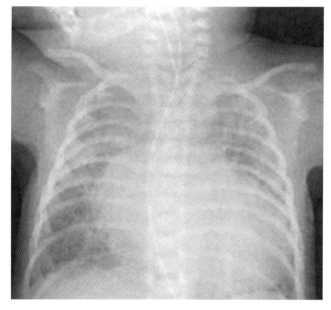

Figure 2.14. Chest x-ray of a newborn with truncus arteriosus. Marked cardiomegaly and significantly increased pulmonary vascular markings are apparent.

Initial Stabilization

1. Maintain O_2 saturation between 75–85% to increase pulmonary vascular resistance and prevent excessive pulmonary blood flow.

2. Prostaglandin E_1 is not necessary unless the infant also has an interrupted aortic arch.

3. Evaluate for 22q11 deletion syndrome (FISH chromosome analysis, immunodeficiency profile, calcium level).

Total Anomalous Pulmonary Venous Return (TAPVR)

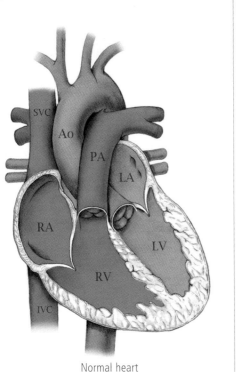

Normal heart

TAPVR affects approximately 1% of all infants with CHD and is characterized by abnormal pulmonary venous drainage directly or indirectly to the right atrium. Pulmonary venous return enters the left atrium through a right-to-left shunt across the foramen ovale or atrial septal defect. Oxygenated blood returning from the lungs mixes with deoxygenated blood returning from the body. Depending on the type of TAPVR, the clinical picture varies from the presentation seen with atrial septal defect, to one characterized by intense cyanosis and profound respiratory distress. Three main types of TAPVR are shown below. A fourth type, mixed, is not shown. Mixed TAPVR involves abnormal pulmonary venous connections to a variety of locations, (vertical or innominate veins, the right atrium or coronary sinus).

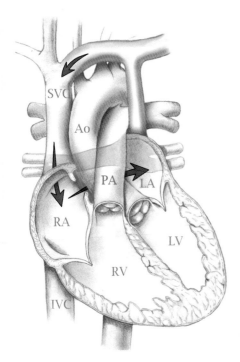

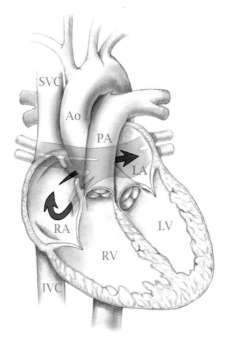

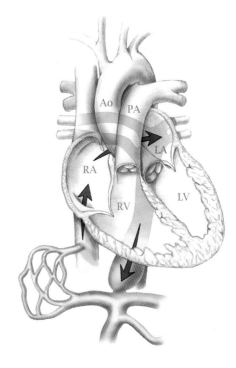

Supracardiac
50% incidence

The pulmonary veins drain to a confluence, which drains a left vertical vein, to the innominate vein, to the right atrium. Affected infants will present with mild to moderate cyanosis.

Cardiac
20% incidence

The pulmonary venous confluence drains to the right atrium via the coronary sinus. Affected infants will present with mild to moderate cyanosis.

Infracardiac
20% incidence

This discussion will focus on infracardiac TAPVR, which is characterized by obstructed pulmonary venous return below the diaphragm. This is the most serious form of TAPVR.

Figure 2.15. Three main types of TAPVR.

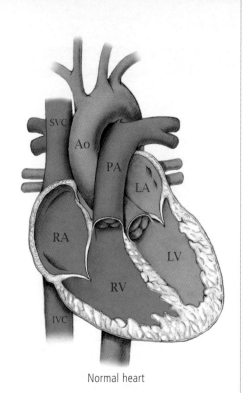

Normal heart

With obstructed total anomalous venous return or connection below the diaphragm via a common collector, oxygenated pulmonary venous blood mixes with deoxygenated systemic venous blood and eventually enters the right atrium as deoxygenated blood. This blood must then shunt right-to-left across the foramen ovale or atrial septal defect into the left atrium, then out the left ventricle to the body. The left ventricular output may be low and the baby may be severely hypoxemic. The pulmonary venous return is obstructed, leading to pulmonary venous congestion, elevated pulmonary vascular resistance, and decreased pulmonary blood flow.

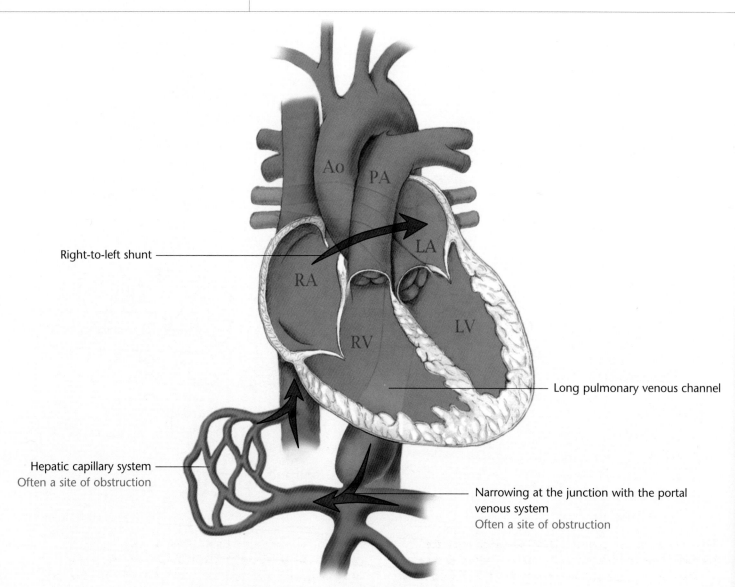

Right-to-left shunt

Long pulmonary venous channel

Hepatic capillary system
Often a site of obstruction

Narrowing at the junction with the portal venous system
Often a site of obstruction

Figure 2.16. Anatomic features of infracardiac TAPVR.

Infracardiac TAPVR Obstructed Below Diaphragm

Sites of obstruction to pulmonary venous blood flow:

♥ Long pulmonary venous channel passes through the diaphragm and is compressed by the diaphragm's action

♥ Narrowing of the channel at the junction with the portal venous system

♥ Hepatic capillary system

♥ Ductus venosus at times

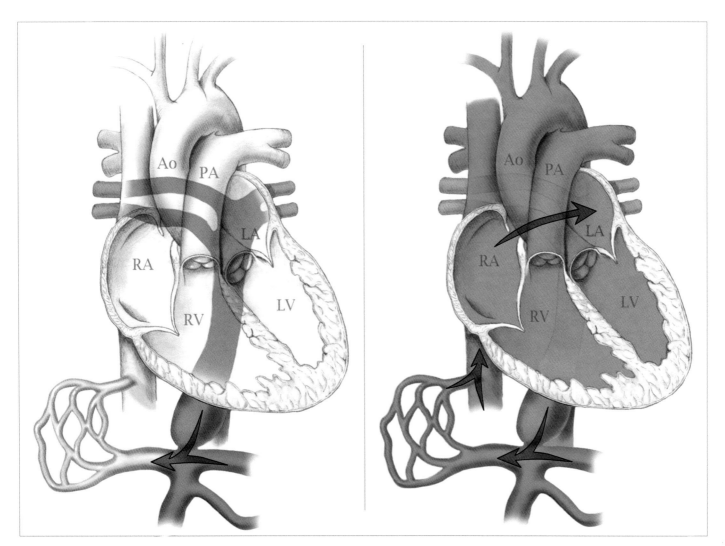

Figure 2.17. Blood flow pattern in TAPVR obstructed below the diaphragm. Oxygenated blood from the pulmonary veins drain via a long pulmonary venous channel through the diaphragm into the portal venous system. Deoxygenated blood in the portal venous system mixes with the oxygenated pulmonary venous blood. Pulmonary venous drainage continues to the hepatic capillary system, the IVC, and into the right atrium. Desaturated blood then shunts right-to-left at the atrial level and through the left heart to reach the aorta.

Infracardiac TAPVR Obstructed Below Diaphragm

Clinical Presentation

♥ Shortly after birth, the infant is profoundly ill.

♥ Obstructed TAPVR — males are affected four times more often than females.

♥ The presentation of obstructed TAPVR mimics severe lung disease and persistent pulmonary hypertension, thus increasing the risk of misdiagnosing the patient with pulmonary disease.

♥ Severe respiratory distress, characterized by tachypnea, retractions, and intense cyanosis, usually requires endotracheal intubation and assisted ventilation.

♥ Obstruction to pulmonary venous return causes severe pulmonary venous hypertension, pulmonary edema, reflex pulmonary venous constriction, and subsequently, pulmonary artery hypertension.

♥ Usually, no murmur is present.

 Neonates may develop a pneumothorax due to the performance of vigorous resuscitation in the setting of abnormal lung compliance.

Chest X-ray

Heart size
The heart size is normal or small.

Pulmonary vasculature
A diffuse reticular pattern of pulmonary edema (hazy lung fields) can be observed.

The condition may be confused with respiratory distress syndrome (RDS) or pneumonia. One distinguishing sign is that the air bronchograms, usually seen with RDS, are not common in TAPVR.

Other
With unobstructed TAPVR the heart size is usually increased.

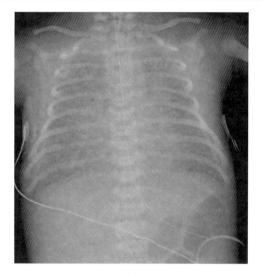

Figure 2.18. Chest x-ray of a neonate with infradiaphragmatic TAPVR. Note the diffuse reticular pulmonary venous pattern secondary to pulmonary edema. The lungs are slightly overinflated. The heart is normal in size.

Initial Stabilization

1. These infants usually require endotracheal intubation and ventilatory support.

2. Provide 100% oxygen.

3. Identify and treat causes of acid-base disturbance, particularly hypotension, hypoxia and hypothermia. In many cases, treatment of the primary cause will resolve metabolic acidosis. If fluid boluses are required and urine output is adequate, consider Ringer's lactate. An inotropic medication (dopamine) may be necessary to treat hypotension.

4. Obtain an echocardiogram early to assist with diagnosis.

5. Emergency corrective surgery, anastomosing the pulmonary venous confluence to the left atrium and ligating the common collector, is usually required.

Ebstein's Anomaly

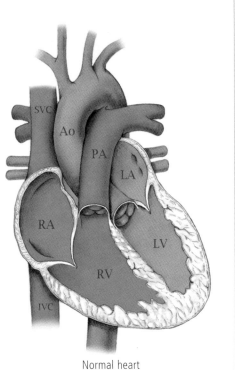

Normal heart

Ebstein's anomaly affects approximately 0.5% of all infants with congenital heart disease. There is an equal male to female distribution. Associated lesions may include a ventricular septal defect and pulmonary stenosis or atresia. Lithium ingestion early in the pregnancy may be associated with the development of Ebstein's anomaly. Supraventricular tachycardia (SVT) occurs in 20% of affected infants. In very severe cases, in-utero cardiac enlargement leads to lung hypoplasia and even fetal death.

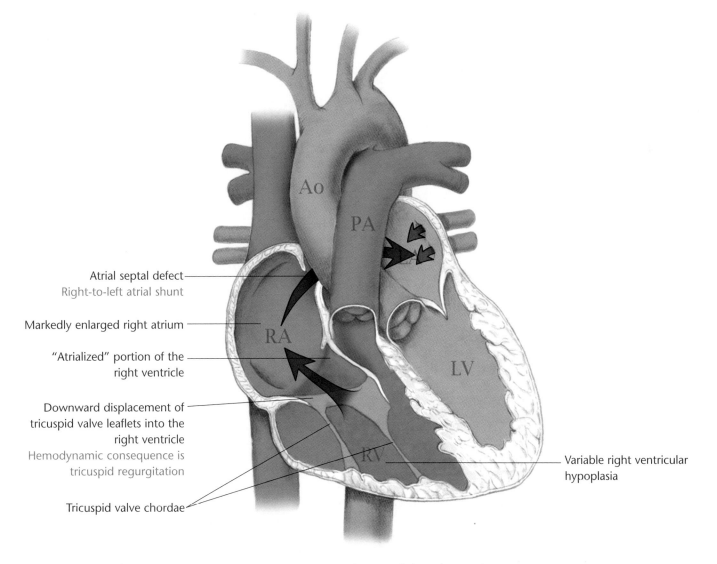

Atrial septal defect
Right-to-left atrial shunt

Markedly enlarged right atrium

"Atrialized" portion of the right ventricle

Downward displacement of tricuspid valve leaflets into the right ventricle
Hemodynamic consequence is tricuspid regurgitation

Tricuspid valve chordae

Variable right ventricular hypoplasia

Figure 2.19. Anatomic features of Ebstein's anomaly.

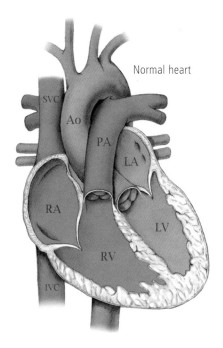

Normal heart

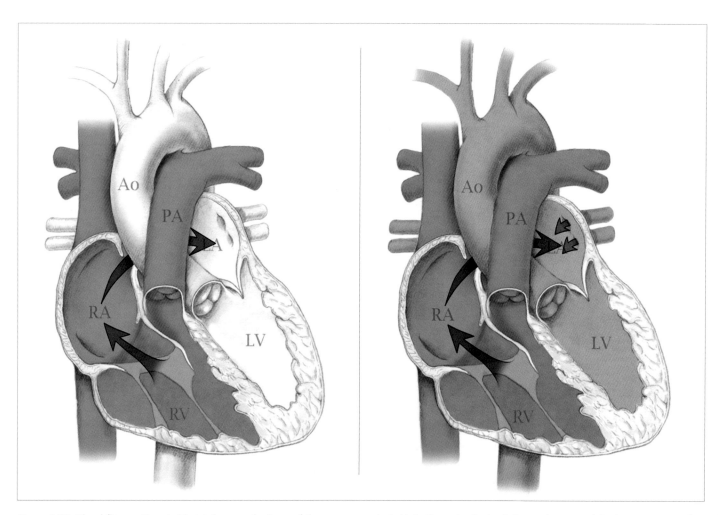

Figure 2.20. Blood flow pattern in Ebstein's anomaly. Some of the blood entering the right ventricle leaks back through the tricuspid valve into the right atrium then shunts right-to-left to the left atrium. Deoxygenated blood mixes with oxygenated blood in the left atrium and is ejected into the systemic circulation and may result in the appearance of cyanosis. Right outflow tract obstruction may be present and, if severe, may result in functional pulmonary atresia.

Ebstein's Anomaly

Ebstein's anomaly

Clinical Presentation

Cyanosis

An affected neonate usually presents with mild to severe cyanosis in the first few days of life. The cyanosis is due to mixing of deoxygenated with oxygenated blood via a right-to-left atrial shunt, which is caused by an elevated right atrial pressure. Because of the abnormal tricuspid valve with significant tricuspid regurgitation, right-to-left atrial shunting occurs, and pulmonary blood flow is decreased. Contraction of the right ventricle usually results in blood flowing backward into the right atrium, with decreased forward flow across the pulmonary valve. In the extreme situation, no blood is ejected across the pulmonary valve (functional pulmonary atresia). The elevated pulmonary vascular resistance seen in neonates compounds the problem. Those with mild cyanosis have little right-to-left shunting at the atrial level and good pulmonary blood flow. Cyanosis usually improves when pulmonary vascular resistance decreases in the post-neonatal period.

Ductal dependence

Neonates with the most severe form of Ebstein's anomaly may be ductal dependent for pulmonary blood flow. If cyanosis is severe and the O_2 saturation is less than 75% while breathing 100% oxygen, a prostaglandin E_1 infusion should be considered. An echocardiogram and evaluation by a pediatric cardiologist should be performed as soon as possible.

Congestive heart failure (CHF)

Symptoms of CHF and hepatomegaly are present in severe cases.

Heart murmur

A gallop rhythm is commonly heard.

A systolic murmur can vary from soft to loud, depending upon the degree of tricuspid regurgitation and pulmonary artery pressure.

Arrhythmias

Supraventricular tachycardia (SVT) occurs in 20% of patients.

Other

In very severe cases, in-utero cardiac enlargement leads to lung hypoplasia.

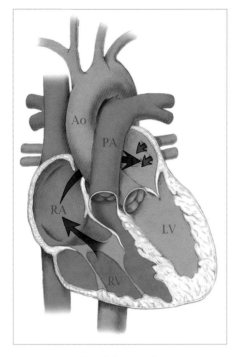

Ebstein's anomaly

Chest X-ray

Heart size and shape

Massive cardiomegaly can be seen if the tricuspid valve is markedly deformed and there is severe regurgitation.

The heart can appear "balloon-shaped."

Pulmonary vascular markings

Decreased pulmonary vascular markings are seen when pulmonary blood flow is decreased.

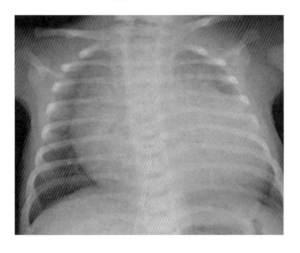
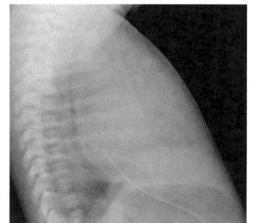

Figure 2.21. Anteroposterior and cross-table lateral radiographs of a one-day old baby with Ebstein's anomaly. Massive cardiomegaly is present (the so-called "wall-to-wall" heart). The pulmonary vasculature is not significantly decreased, as it usually is. An umbilical venous catheter is present with its tip in the right atrium.

Initial Stabilization

1. Extreme forms of Ebstein's may be ductal dependent. If the O_2 saturation is < 75%, consider starting a prostaglandin E_1 infusion.

2. Place the infant on oxygen to help lower the pulmonary vascular resistance (PVR) and improve pulmonary blood flow.

3. Inotropes may be necessary to treat hypotension and congestive heart failure.

4. Correct metabolic acidosis to reverse the negative effect of acidosis on the pulmonary vasculature.

5. Treat SVT if it occurs.

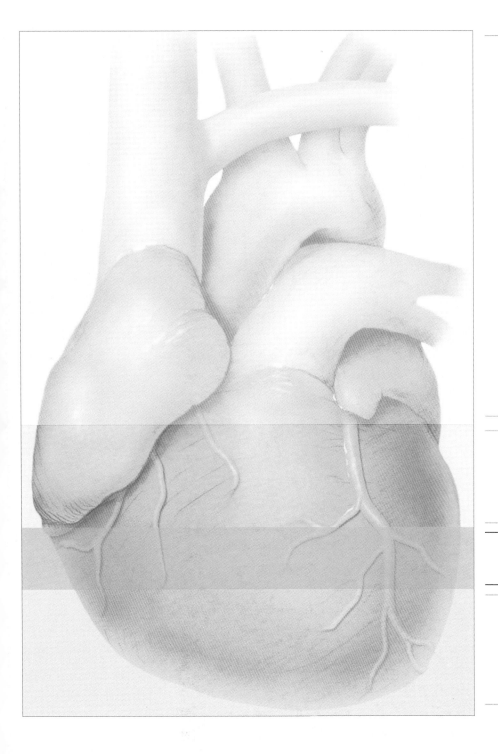

All other congenital heart
defects — 58%

Cyanotic CHD, not ductal
dependent — 15%

**Transposition of the
great arteries — 5%**

Tricuspid atresia — 1–3%

**Pulmonary atresia — <1%
(with IVS)**

Tetralogy with severe PS or atresia

Severe Ebstein's

Left outflow tract CHD, ductal
dependent for systemic blood
flow — 18%

Cyanotic CHD
Ductal dependent for PBF

Underlying Concepts

The previous discussion on cyanotic CHD focused on lesions that are usually not dependent on the ductus arteriosus for pulmonary blood flow. This next section will review cyanotic congenital heart lesions that *are dependent* on the ductus arteriosus for pulmonary blood flow or to improve intercirculatory mixing as in transposition of the great arteries.

- When blood flow to the lungs is reduced because of severe narrowing or atresia of the pulmonary outflow tract, blood must enter the lungs via an aorta-to-pulmonary artery shunt. This is typically through a left-to-right shunt via the patent ductus arteriosus.

- As the ductus arteriosus closes in left-to-right ductal dependent lesions, blood flow to the body remains adequate, but blood flow to the lungs is reduced. When a smaller amount of blood enters the lungs, a smaller amount of red or oxygenated blood returns from the lungs. The proportion of blue blood to red blood ejected through the aorta increases and the infant will appear cyanotic. Once the ductus is re-opened with a prostaglandin E_1 infusion, pulmonary blood flow improves; the proportion of red blood to blue blood increases and cyanosis improves.

- With transposition of the great arteries (TGA), oxygenated blood returning to the left atrium is ejected by the left ventricle back to the lungs (i.e., blood flow to the lungs is not decreased). The aorta ejects deoxygenated right ventricular blood to the systemic circulation. Good mixing between the right and left hearts is essential so that oxygenated blood can be ejected to the systemic circulation. When the ductus is re-opened with a prostaglandin E_1 infusion, mixing can occur due to bidirectional ductal shunting. In addition, atrial mixing may improve.

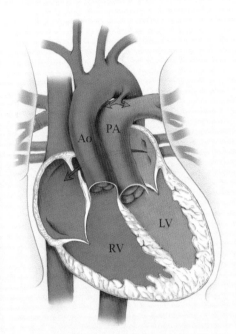

Transposition of the great arteries

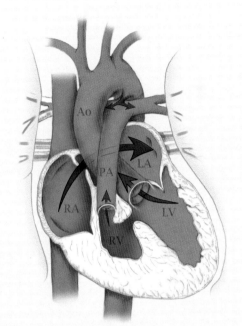

Tricuspid atresia

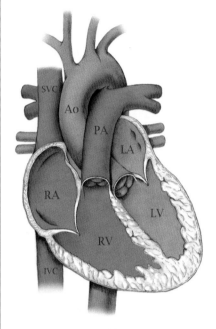

Normal heart

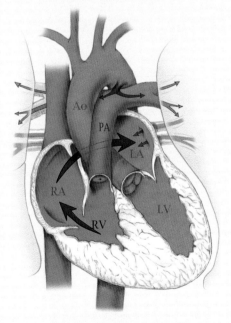

Pulmonary atresia with intact
ventricular septum

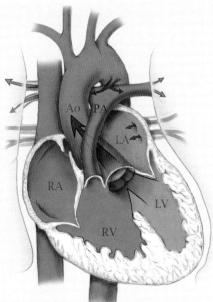
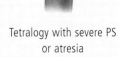

Tetralogy with severe PS
or atresia

Figure 2.22. Comparative illustrations of the CHD lesions that are ductal dependent for
pulmonary blood flow.

The Ductus Arteriosus

In utero, the placenta, not the lung, is the site of gas exchange. In the fetus, most of the blood entering the right ventricle bypasses the lungs by flowing through the ductus arteriosus, a connection between the pulmonary artery and aorta. The ductus is lined with smooth muscle and functionally closes within the first few hours to days after birth.

One factor contributing to closure of the ductus is vasoconstriction in response to an increase in arterial oxygenation, which occurs when the lungs take over gas exchange after birth. Complete anatomic closure of the ductus usually occurs between 2 and 4 weeks of life.

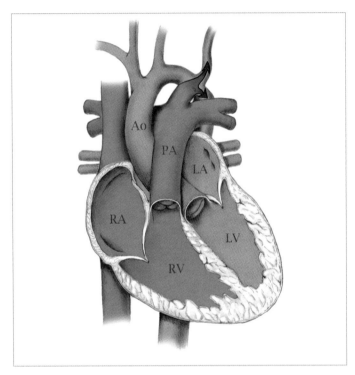

Figure 2.23. Illustration demonstrating a right-to-left shunt at the ductus arteriosus. Deoxygenated blood flows into the pulmonary artery, where variable amounts of blood shunt through the ductus arteriosus to the aorta.

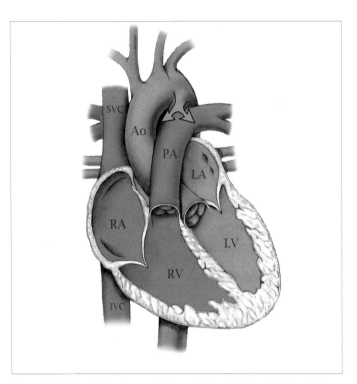

Figure 2.24. Illustration demonstrating a left-to-right shunt at the ductus arteriosus. Oxygenated blood flows through the aorta, with variable amounts of blood shunting through the ductus arteriosus into the pulmonary arteries and lungs.

What is Ductal Dependence?

At times, blood flow to the lungs or to the systemic circulation may be limited by structural abnormalities in the heart. Neonates with severe left heart obstruction (coarctation, critical aortic stenosis, interrupted aortic arch, hypoplastic left ventricle) depend on a right-to-left shunt through the ductus arteriosus for systemic circulation. Ductal closure results in impaired systemic perfusion, often in conjunction with heart failure, and if left untreated, death.

Neonates with right ventricular outflow tract obstruction, tricuspid atresia with pulmonary stenosis, pulmonary atresia with intact ventricular septum, critical PS, tetralogy with severe PS or atresia, and infants with transposition of the great arteries, depend on a left-to-right shunt through the ductus arteriosus for pulmonary circulation. Without this shunt, they would suffer inadequate pulmonary blood flow and severe life-threatening hypoxemia, which would, if left untreated, lead to death.

Pharmacology The Ductus Arteriosus

Prostaglandin E$_1$ (Alprostadil, Prostin, PGE$_1$)

Indications

To open or maintain patency of the ductus arteriosus.

Action

Causes vasodilation by direct effect on the smooth muscle in the ductus arteriosus and usually works within minutes to hours of beginning the medication.

Treatment Goals

Improve oxygen saturation in lesions dependent on the ductus for pulmonary blood flow.

Improve blood pressure and perfusion in lesions dependent on the ductus for systemic blood flow.

Dose

1. Begin at 0.05 to 0.1 micrograms/kilogram/minute.

2. May increase to 0.2 to 0.4 mcg/kg/minute if there is no response.

3. *NICU Management*: Once the ductus is widely open, the pediatric cardiologist may request a gradual decrease in dose to 0.01 to 0.03 mcg/kg/minute.

Expected response

Increase in arterial PO$_2$ or increase in blood pressure.

Improvement in metabolic acidosis as a result of improving perfusion or hypoxia.

Infusion Rules

Infuse via a separate IV site.

PGE$_1$ is compatible in D5W, D10W or normal saline but is not compatible with other medications.

PGE$_1$ has a very short half-life and therefore must be administered as a continuous drip infusion.

Once the ductus is widely open, use the lowest dose possible to minimize side effects.

Side Effects

Respiratory (usually dose dependent)

Respiratory depression or apnea may occur.

Apnea is usually seen within the first few hours of infusion.

Increased incidence of apnea is associated with body weight less than 2 kilograms.

 Be prepared to support ventilation.

Cardiovascular

Flushing, hypotension, bradycardia, tachycardia

CNS

Irritability, jitteriness, seizure-like activity, fever

Endocrine

Hypocalcemia and hypoglycemia

Gastrointestinal

Stimulates intestinal smooth muscle and may cause diarrhea

Hematologic

Inhibits platelet aggregation, monitor for bleeding

This icon represents a PGE$_1$ infusion.

Transposition of the Great Arteries (TGA)

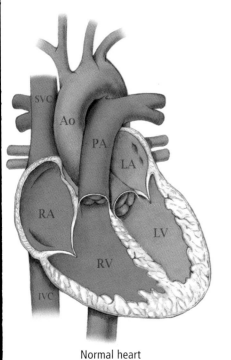

Normal heart

TGA affects approximately 5% of all infants with CHD. The male to female ratio is 3 to 1. As the name suggests, the great arteries are transposed relative to the ventricle. The aorta arises anteriorly from the right ventricle and ejects deoxygenated blood to the body; the pulmonary artery arises posteriorly from the left ventricle and recirculates oxygenated blood to the lungs. This circulation pattern is parallel, meaning the majority of blood ejected from a ventricle is recirculated back to that same ventricle. In order for oxygenated blood to reach the systemic circulation, mixing of the pulmonary and systemic venous return must occur at one or more of three locations: a patent foramen ovale (PFO) or atrial septal defect (ASD), a ventricular septal defect (VSD), or a patent ductus arteriosus (PDA). A VSD is present in approximately 40–45% of patients.

Mixing of pulmonary and systemic circulations must occur at the ductal, atrial, and/or ventricular level.

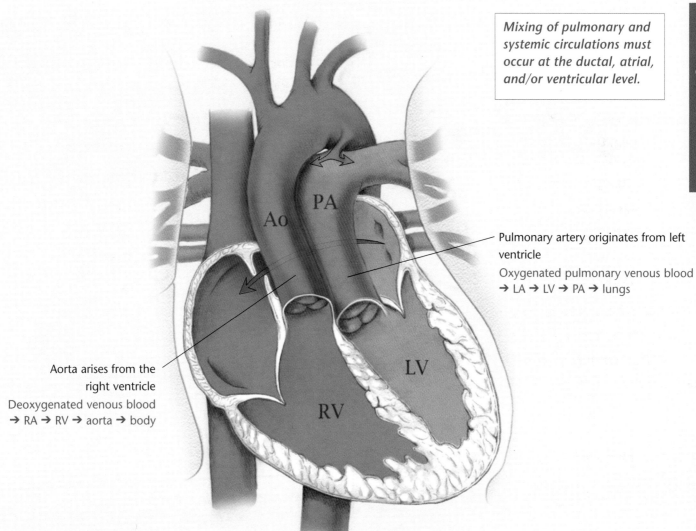

Pulmonary artery originates from left ventricle

Oxygenated pulmonary venous blood
➔ LA ➔ LV ➔ PA ➔ lungs

Aorta arises from the right ventricle
Deoxygenated venous blood
➔ RA ➔ RV ➔ aorta ➔ body

Figure 2.25. Anatomic features of TGA.

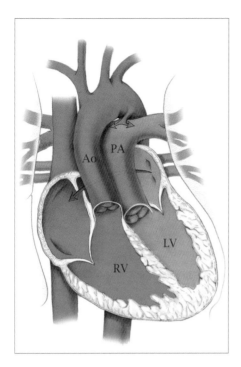

Figure 2.26. TGA with a closing ductus arteriosus. In the absence of a VSD and/or good atrial mixing, oxygenated blood will re-circulate to the lungs and deoxygenated blood will circulate systemically.

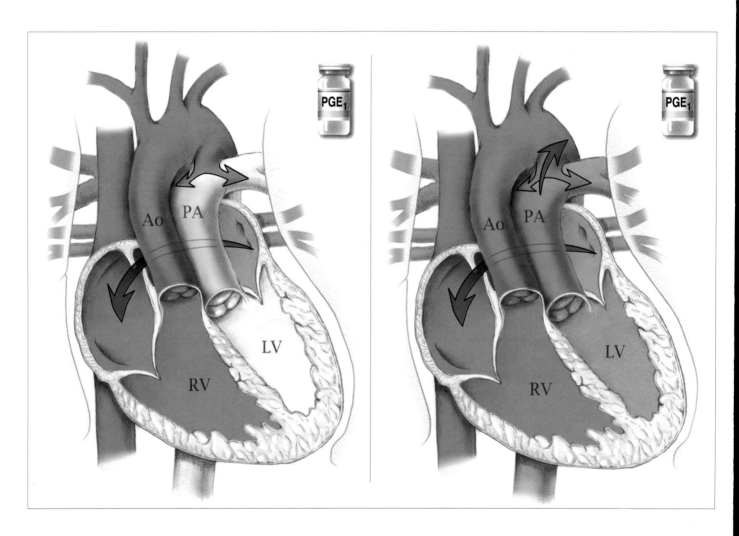

Figure 2.27. Pattern of blood flow seen when PGE₁ re-establishes ductal patency. Improved pulmonary blood flow will help raise the left atrial pressure and improve the left-to-right atrial shunt. This illustration shows blood shunting both right to left and left to right through the ductus arteriosus. This may result in reverse differential cyanosis where the saturation or PO_2 in the right hand is lower than the saturation or PO_2 in the lower body.

Transposition of the Great Arteries (TGA)

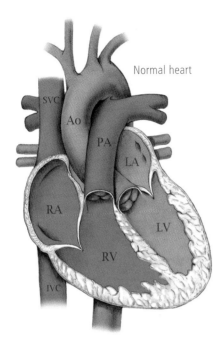

Normal heart

Clinical Presentation

For neonates with TGA and an *intact ventricular septum*, the size of the atrial septal defect influences the degree of mixing of the pulmonary and systemic circulation and thus, the severity of the cyanosis. If the defect is small, moderate to severe cyanosis is noted at birth or shortly thereafter. Arterial PO_2 may be as low as 15 to 25 mmHg. Severe hypoxemia leads to anaerobic glycolysis, severe acidemia, and if not reversed, death.

Neonates with TGA and a sizeable *ventricular septal defect* may have increased pulmonary blood flow and mild cyanosis with crying. Congestive heart failure — tachypnea, tachycardia, hepatomegaly, and a loud murmur — develop by the second to sixth week of life. This discussion, however, will focus on neonates who are acutely ill with TGA, those with an intact ventricular septum.

Athough tachypneic and cyanotic, the neonate usually appears quite comfortable. With progressive hypoxemia and the development of metabolic acidosis, however, an increase in respiratory effort can be observed. This observation is important for differentiating between pulmonary and cardiac disease. With pulmonary disease, neonates exhibiting a high degree of hypoxemia (PO_2 between 15 to 25 mm Hg) usually present with more pronounced respiratory distress, characterized by retractions, dyspnea, and elevated arterial PCO_2. With TGA, the PCO_2 is usually less than 45 (the effect of hyperventilation with normal lung compliance), and there may be evidence of metabolic acidosis (low pH, normal or low pCO_2).

Heart sounds

The S2 is single and loud, secondary to a loud A2 component, as the aortic valve is anterior to the pulmonary valve.

Variable murmur

If the ventricular septum is intact, there is often no murmur. A systolic murmur may be heard in neonates with a VSD. If associated pulmonary stenosis is present, a systolic ejection murmur is usually heard.

Transposition of the Great Arteries (TGA)

Pre- and post-ductal saturation

Evaluation of pre- and post-ductal saturation will help differentiate TGA from persistent pulmonary hypertension of the newborn (PPHN), which may present in a similar manner. With PPHN, the pre-ductal, right subclavian artery (right hand) saturation will be higher than the post-ductal (leg) saturation, if there is a large right-to-left ductal shunt, (providing the baby is not severely hypoxemic and there is no significant right-to-left atrial shunt).

Neonates with a large PDA and TGA may have a *reverse differential cyanosis* (e.g., the right arm saturation will be lower than the leg saturation). The mechanism for this saturation pattern is as follows: oxygenated, saturated blood flows from the lungs to the LA, LV, PA, through the ductus arteriosus and distal aorta, to the body, resulting in relatively high saturation values detected by an oximeter located on the foot. Conversely, deoxygenated, desaturated systemic venous blood flows to the RA, RV, and out the aorta. Deoxygenated blood therefore supplies the right subclavian artery (pre-ductal), resulting in relatively low saturation values detected by an oximeter located on the right hand. This pattern is the opposite of the saturation pattern seen in PPHN and is therefore an important observation.

Chest X-ray

Heart size
Mild cardiomegaly is usually present.

Shape
A characteristic oval or egg-shaped appearance ("egg on a string") of the heart is due to a narrow mediastinum, caused by a small thymus and alignment of the great vessels over each other.

Pulmonary vascular markings
Increased pulmonary vascular markings are secondary to increased pulmonary blood flow.

 Right ventricular blood is ejected directly into the aorta. A central venous catheter tip positioned at the IVC/RA junction must be carefully handled to prevent emboli from reaching the systemic circulation.

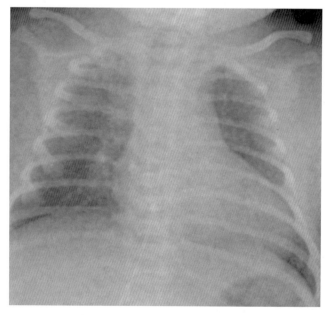

Figure 2.28. Chest x-ray of a neonate with TGA. Note the abnormal heart shape and increased pulmonary vascular markings.

Transposition of the Great Arteries (TGA)

Initial Stabilization

Treatment is aimed at establishing ductal patency, and if indicated, improving mixing at the atrial level.

1. Improve pulmonary blood flow. Blood shunts down a pressure gradient. In TGA, shunting from the left atrium to the right atrium requires adequate pulmonary venous return. The following measures help improve pulmonary blood flow and subsequently improve pulmonary venous return:

   • Provide O_2 to decrease pulmonary vascular resistance, which will encourage more blood to enter the lungs.

   • Start PGE_1 to open the ductus arteriosus and allow the following pattern of blood flow:

   > Aorta ➜ **deoxygenated blood** shunts through the ductus arteriosus ➜ pulmonary artery ➜ lungs ➜ **oxygenated blood** returns to the left atrium ➜ shunts left-to-right across the foramen ovale or ASD to the right atrium ➜ right ventricle ➜ aorta ➜ to descending aorta and ductus arteriosus again.

2. Identify and treat causes of metabolic acidosis.

3. Evaluate right arm and leg saturation. A widely patent ductus arteriosus may cause the right arm saturation (and brain oxygenation) to be lower than the systemic saturation (*reverse differential cyanosis*). Keep the right arm saturation >75%.

4. Persistent severe hypoxemia, after establishing a patent ductus arteriosus, indicates restricted atrial communication and subsequent poor mixing of oxygenated with deoxygenated blood. A Rashkind balloon atrial septostomy procedure is indicated.

Rashkind balloon atrial septostomy

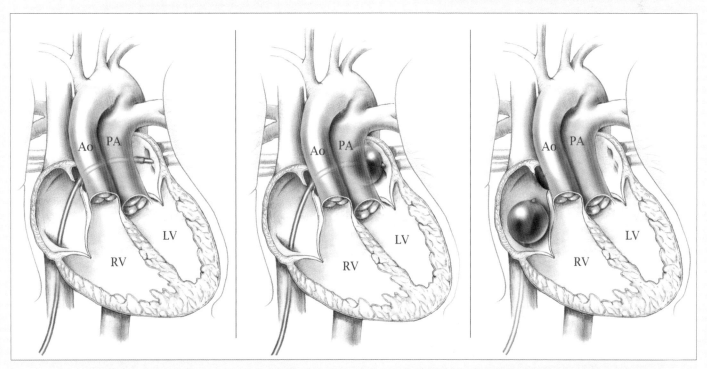

Figure 2.29. A balloon-tipped catheter is inserted into the left atrium through the patent foramen ovale. The balloon is inflated and then rapidly pulled back into the right atrium using echocardiographic or x-ray guidance. The third illustration shows the atrial septal defect that is created with this procedure.

Type 1

TAtr with normally related great arteries is observed in 70% of cases.

Type 2

TAtr with transposition of the great arteries occurs in 30% of cases.

Patients with TAtr and TGA have increased pulmonary blood flow. Therefore cyanosis is less severe, and pulmonary overcirculation with CHF is likely to develop. Other associated lesions include coarctation of the aorta (shown) and interrupted aortic arch.

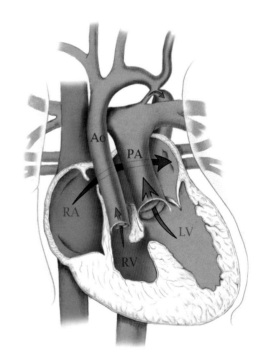

Figure 2.30. TAtr with TGA and coarctation of the aorta.

Tricuspid Atresia (TAtr)

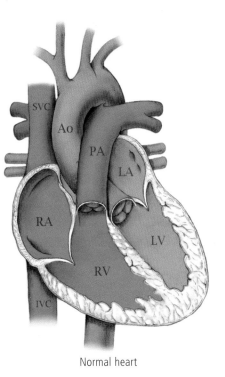

Normal heart

TAtr affects approximately 1–3% of all infants with CHD. Males and females are equally affected unless there is an associated TGA, in which case males are more frequently affected.

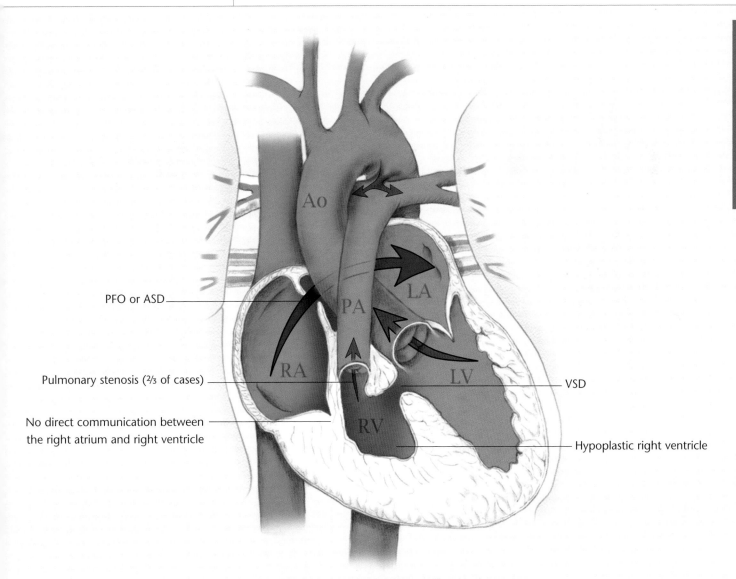

PFO or ASD

Pulmonary stenosis (⅔ of cases)

No direct communication between the right atrium and right ventricle

VSD

Hypoplastic right ventricle

Figure 2.31. Anatomic features of TAtr with normally related great arteries.

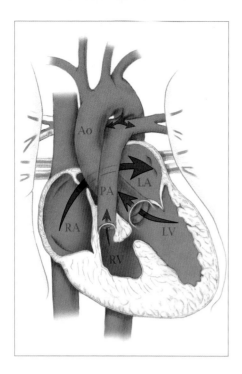

Figure 2.32. TAtr with a closing ductus arteriosus. The degree of pulmonary stenosis will influence whether this lesion is ductal dependent. This illustration shows moderate pulmonary stenosis and ductal dependency.

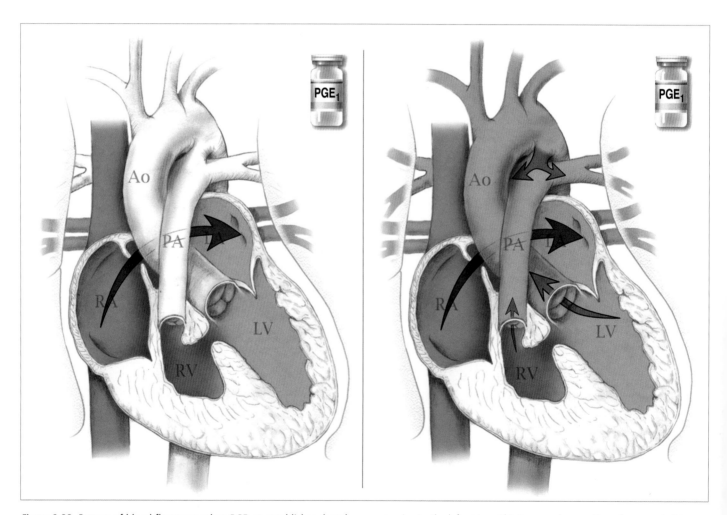

Figure 2.33. Pattern of blood flow seen when PGE$_1$ re-establishes ductal patency. Blood will shunt left-to-right (aorta to pulmonary) through the ductus arteriosus and result in a larger proportion of oxygenated blood returning to the left atrium. This increased proportion of oxygenated to deoxygenated blood will help improve the PO$_2$ of blood entering the systemic circulation.

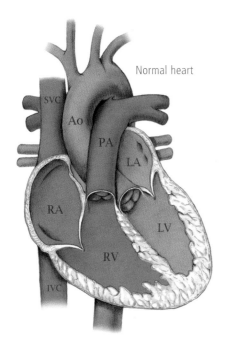

Normal heart

Tricuspid Atresia (TAtr)

This discussion focuses on the presentation and stabilization of neonates with TAtr who have normally related great arteries. There is no direct communication between the right atrium and right ventricle. The right ventricle is hypoplastic. Blood entering the right atrium must shunt across the patent foramen ovale or ASD to the left atrium. Blood entering the left ventricle is ejected into the aorta and through a VSD to the small right ventricle, which gives rise to the pulmonary artery. As many as two-thirds of patients with TA have a component of pulmonary stenosis, which ranges from mild to complete atresia. The size of the VSD also contributes to adequacy of pulmonary blood flow. Neonates with TAtr with normally related great arteries and significant pulmonary stenosis are ductal dependent for pulmonary blood flow.

Clinical Presentation

Neonates usually present in the first week of life with cyanosis, tachypnea, and poor feeding.

Cyanosis

Hypoxemia worsens with increased degrees of pulmonary stenosis and with restriction of left-to-right blood flow at the level of the VSD.

Thrill

If the VSD is restrictive, a thrill might be present.

Heart sounds

The first heart sound is single and accentuated.

The second heart sound is usually single.

Murmur

A grade 2–3/6 regurgitant VSD murmur may be heard at the LLSB.

A PS murmur may be heard if pulmonary stenosis is present.

A continuous PDA murmur may be present.

Pulses

Brachial and femoral pulses can be felt, unless coarctation is present, in which case femoral pulses may be difficult to feel. Coarctation is usually associated with tricuspid atresia and transposed rather than normally related great vessels.

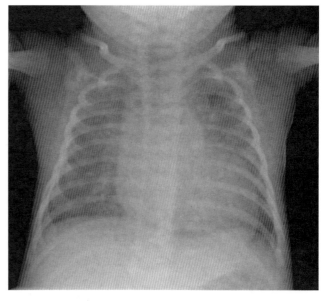

Figure 2.34. TAtr with a closing ductus arteriosus.

Chest X-ray

Heart size
The heart size is normal to slightly increased.

Shape
The heart may appear globular or "boot shaped," as in TOF, because of the concave main PA segment.

Pulmonary vasculature
Decreased pulmonary vascular markings are seen in 80% of patients.

Increased pulmonary vascular markings are seen with TAtr and TGA or a large VSD and no associated pulmonary stenosis.

Other
Incidence of right aortic arch is 3–8%.

Tricuspid Atresia (TAtr)

Figure 2.35. Chest x-ray of a neonate with tricuspid atresia, pulmonary stenosis and on a PGE$_1$ infusion. Mild cardiomegaly with increased pulmonary vascular markings are apparent.

Initial Stabilization

Treatment is aimed at improving pulmonary blood flow and reversing the effects of severe hypoxemia.

The approach to cyanotic neonates with suspected CHD remains the same as discussed previously:

1. Begin 100% oxygen to improve systemic oxygenation and decrease pulmonary vascular resistance.

2. If the O$_2$ saturation remains below 75% on 100% oxygen, begin a PGE$_1$ infusion to maintain ductal patency.

3. Maintain O$_2$ saturation > 75%.

4. Evaluate and treat underlying causes of acidosis.

Pulmonary Atresia (PAtr with IVS)

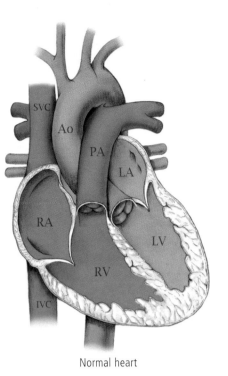

Normal heart

Pulmonary atresia (PAtr) with intact ventricular septum (IVS) affects approximately 1% of infants with CHD and is characterized by an atretic pulmonary valve, and a hypertrophied, hypoplastic right ventricle. Pulmonary blood flow is dependent upon a patent ductus arteriosus. The high right ventricular pressure leads to anomalies of the coronary circulation in 30–60% of patients.

Because of the right ventricular outflow tract obstruction, blood from the right ventricle leaks back through the tricuspid valve to the right atrium, where it shunts right to left through a patent foramen ovale or atrial septal defect, to the left atrium. Some neonates have significant, problematic tricuspid regurgitation.

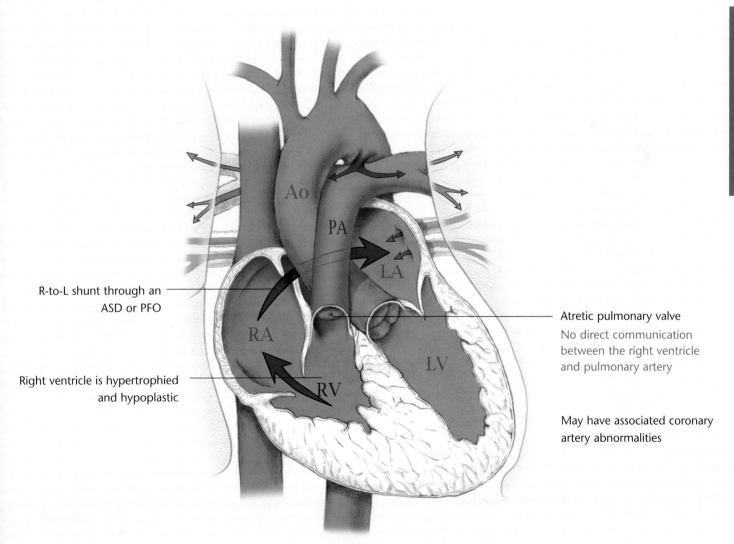

R-to-L shunt through an ASD or PFO

Atretic pulmonary valve

No direct communication between the right ventricle and pulmonary artery

Right ventricle is hypertrophied and hypoplastic

May have associated coronary artery abnormalities

Figure 2.36. Anatomic features of PAtr with intact ventricular septum (IVS).

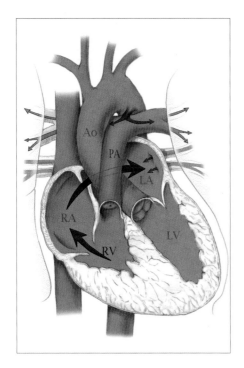

Figure 2.37. PAtr with a closing ductus arteriosus. Pulmonary blood flow decreases significantly with closure of the ductus arteriosus, resulting in severe hypoxemia.

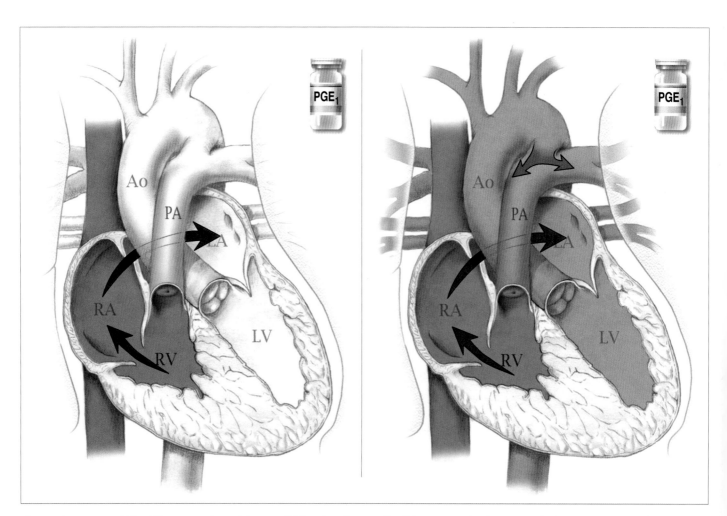

Figure 2.38. Pattern of blood flow seen when PGE₁ re-establishes ductal patency. In order to perfuse the lungs, blood must shunt left to right from the aorta to the pulmonary artery. Once the ductus is re-opened, cyanosis will still be apparent but hypoxemia should lessen because of the increased proportion of oxygenated to deoxygenated blood that is ejected into the aorta.

Tetralogy of Fallot with Pulmonary Atresia

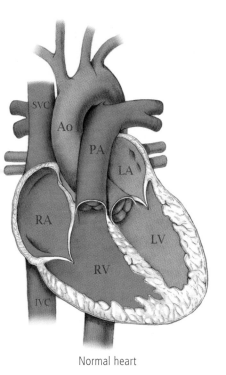

Normal heart

Tetralogy of Fallot with pulmonary atresia and pulmonary atresia with intact ventricular septum present very similarly and will therefore be discussed together. Despite their superficial similarities however, their anatomy, associated features, timing of treatment, and long-term prognosis are quite different.

This is the most extreme form of tetralogy of Fallot (TOF). All blood entering the right and left ventricles is ejected into the overriding aorta. The desaturated right ventricular blood and the limited volume of oxygenated blood returning from the lungs are both ejected into the aorta, resulting in hypoxemia.

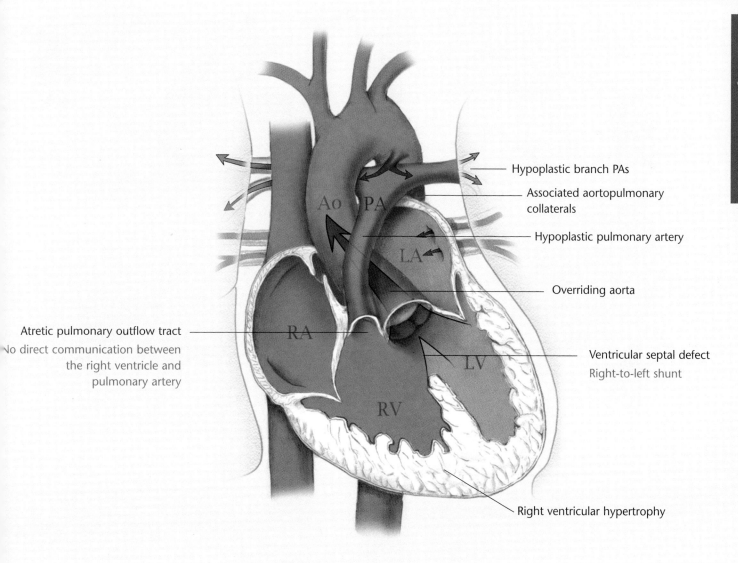

Hypoplastic branch PAs

Associated aortopulmonary collaterals

Hypoplastic pulmonary artery

Overriding aorta

Atretic pulmonary outflow tract
No direct communication between the right ventricle and pulmonary artery

Ventricular septal defect
Right-to-left shunt

Right ventricular hypertrophy

Figure 2.39. Anatomic features of TOF with pulmonary atresia.

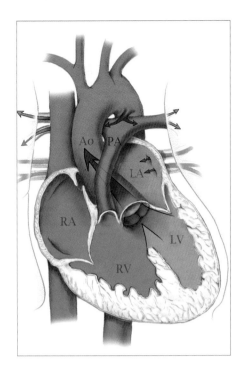

Figure 2.40. TOF with PAtr with a closing ductus arteriosus. Pulmonary blood flow decreases significantly with closure of the ductus arteriosus. Deoxygenated and oxygenated blood that mixes at the VSD is ejected into the aorta and systemic circulation, resulting in the appearance of cyanosis.

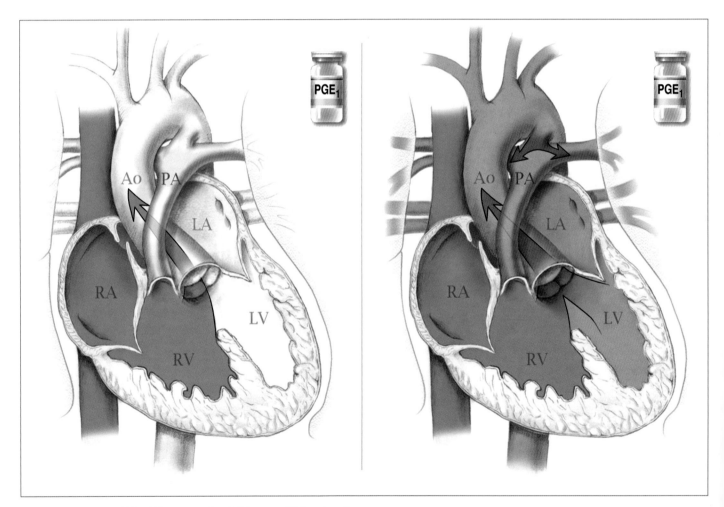

Figure 2.41. Pattern of blood flow seen when PGE$_1$ re-establishes ductal patency. Blood must shunt left-to-right from the aorta to the pulmonary artery. Once the ductus is re-opened, hypoxemia and cyanosis should decrease because of the increased proportion of oxygenated to deoxygenated blood.

PAtr with IVS and TOF with PAtr

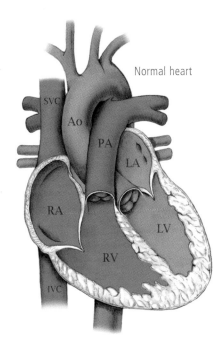

Normal heart

Clinical Presentation

Pulmonary atresia with intact ventricular septum and TOF with pulmonary atresia

These infants usually present at birth with varying degrees of cyanosis and respiratory distress. As the ductus arteriosus closes, affected neonates become intensely cyanotic.

Cyanosis

Variable cyanosis is apparent from birth; it worsens dramatically with closure of the ductus arteriosus.

Heart sounds

The second heart sound is single because of absence of the P2 component.

Murmur

Pulmonary atresia with intact ventricular septum: If a heart murmur is present, it will be secondary to tricuspid regurgitation and/or a patent ductus arteriosus.

TOF with pulmonary atresia: If a heart murmur is present, it will be secondary to a patent ductus arteriosus or aortopulmonary collaterals.

Chest X-ray

Heart size

Pulmonary atresia with intact ventricular septum:
The heart size is variably enlarged, reflecting
enlargement of the right atrium and left ventricle.

TOF with pulmonary atresia: The heart size is small
or normal.

Shape

TOF with pulmonary atresia: Boot-shaped
appearance is secondary to hypoplasia of the
pulmonary artery segment and right ventricular
hypertrophy.

Pulmonary vasculature

Decreased pulmonary vascular markings are
characteristic of both pulmonary atresia with IVS
and TOF with pulmonary atresia.

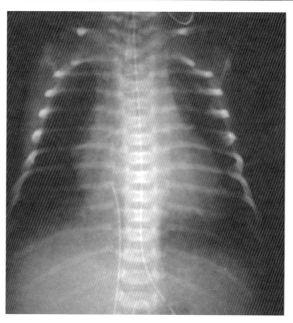

Figure 2.42. Chest x-ray of a term neonate with pulmonary atresia.
Pulmonary vascular markings are decreased and the heart is moderately
enlarged. The infant is intubated and the lungs are hyperinflated.

Initial Stabilization

Pulmonary atresia with intact ventricular septum and TOF with pulmonary atresia

The stabilization principles are the same for these
two heart lesions. Treatment is aimed at improving
pulmonary blood flow and reversing the effects of
severe hypoxemia. The approach to cyanotic
neonates with suspected congenital heart disease
remains the same as discussed previously:

1. Begin 100% oxygen to improve systemic
   oxygenation and decrease pulmonary vascular
   resistance.

2. Begin an infusion of PGE_1 to re-establish and
   maintain ductal patency.

3. Maintain O_2 saturation > 75%.

4. Evaluate and treat underlying causes of acidosis.

 *Because of the right-to-left shunt at either the
atrial or ventricular level, use extra caution with
central venous catheters to prevent emboli from
reaching the systemic circulation.*

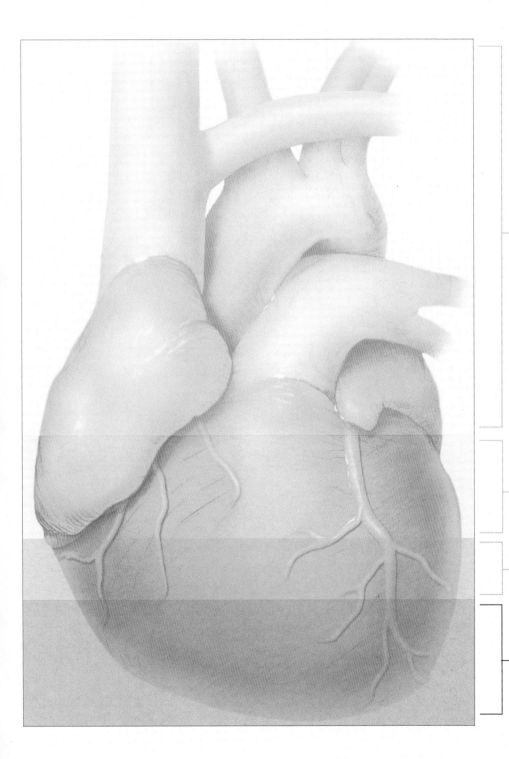

All other congenital heart defects — 58%

Cyanotic CHD, not ductal dependent — 15%

Cyanotic CHD, ductal dependent for pulmonary blood flow — 9%

Coarctation of the aorta — 8–10%
Critical aortic stenosis — 3–6%
Interrupted aortic arch — 1%
Hypoplastic left heart syndrome — 1%

Left outflow tract CHD
Ductal dependent for SBF

Underlying Concepts

- Systemic blood flow (body, brain, and heart muscle itself via the coronary circulation) may be reduced because of either of the following:

  - Anatomic narrowing (coarctation) or interruption of the aortic arch; or

  - Severe obstruction at the aortic or mitral valve level, as seen with critical aortic stenosis or hypoplastic left heart syndrome.

- With severe left heart obstructive lesions, systemic perfusion is dependent upon a *right-to-left* ductal shunt. As the ductus arteriosus closes, systemic blood flow is severely reduced and leads to congestive heart failure, and in some cases, shock.

- When the ductus is re-opened with a prostaglandin E_1 infusion, blood flows from the pulmonary artery to the aorta — a right-to-left ductal shunt. The patient may exhibit varying degrees of cyanosis depending on the underlying cardiac abnormality.

- In some cases, blood flow to the brain and coronary circulation is dependent on blood that flows from the ductus retrograde around the arch to the head and neck vessels and ascending aorta.

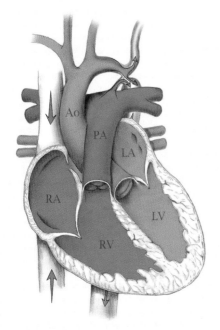

Coarctation of the aorta

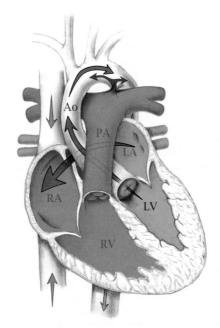

Critical aortic valve stenosis

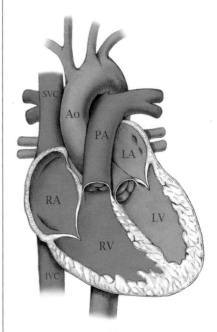

Normal heart

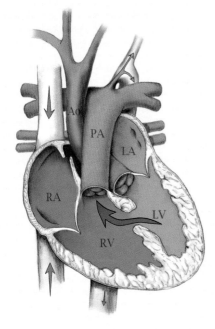

Interrupted aortic arch

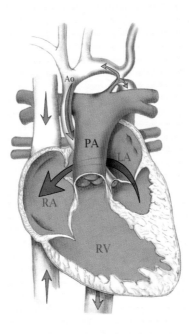

Hypoplastic left heart syndrome

Figure 2.43. Comparative illustrations of the left outflow tract obstructive lesions discussed in this section.

Coarctation of the Aorta (COA)

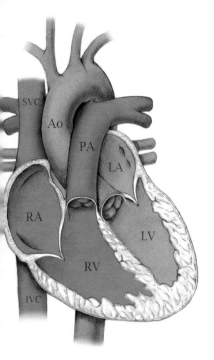

Normal heart

COA accounts for 8–10% of all cases of CHD and is seen twice as often in males as in females; the incidence in Turner's syndrome, which affects only females, is 30 percent. COA is characterized by a narrowed aortic lumen, most often in the aorta across from the ductus arteriosus. There is wide variation in the appearance of the aorta, ranging from short discrete narrowing to long segment stenosis. The transverse arch may be hypoplastic and associated cardiac defects, including a bicuspid aortic valve, mitral valve abnormalities, and VSDs, are common.

When the ductus is open, blood shunts right to left (PA to Ao). Ductal tissue often extends into the area of coarctation; with ductal closure, the narrowing may become severe. In severe COA, CHF results from the inability of the left ventricle to pump against the narrowed aorta. In extreme cases, signs of shock become apparent.

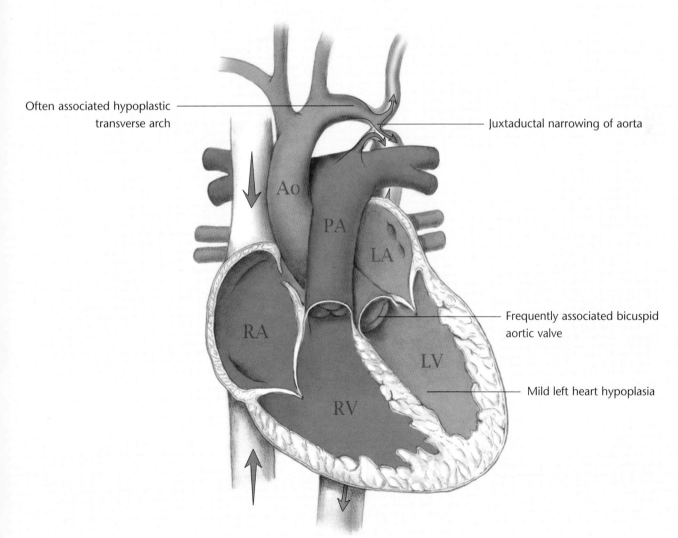

Often associated hypoplastic transverse arch

Juxtaductal narrowing of aorta

Frequently associated bicuspid aortic valve

Mild left heart hypoplasia

Left outflow tract CHD
Ductal dependent for SBF

Figure 2.4. Anatomic features of COA.

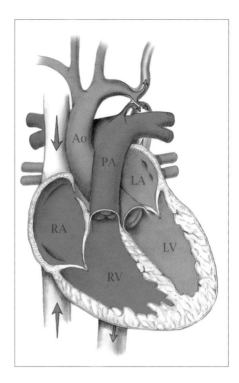

Figure 2.45. COA with a closing ductus arteriosus. As the ductus closes, the area of coarctation narrows and results in decreased systemic blood flow. In severe cases, CHF results from decreased left ventricular function as the heart attempts to pump against the narrowed aorta. With ductal closure, severe coarctation leads to the development of shock and tissue hypoxia.

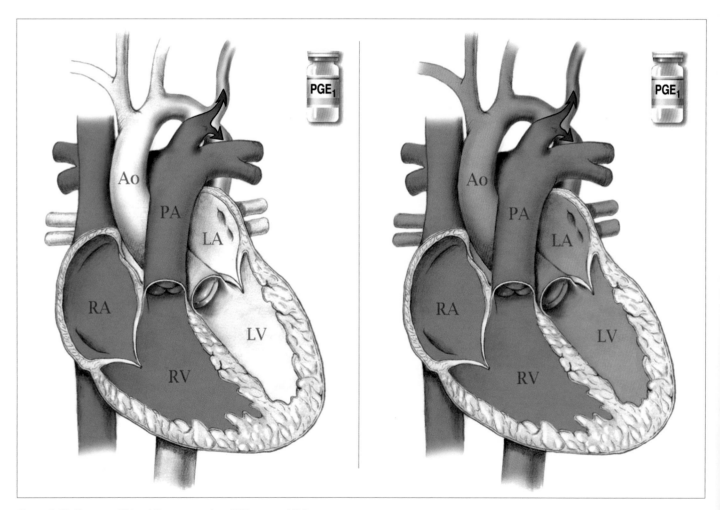

Figure 2.46. Pattern of blood flow seen when PGE_1 re-establishes ductal patency. Blood will shunt right to left from the pulmonary artery to the aorta and then into the systemic circulation.

Critical Aortic Valve Stenosis (AS)

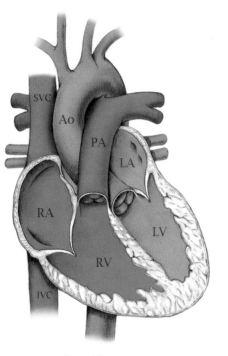

Normal heart

AS accounts for approximately 3–6% of all cases of CHD, with males affected four times more often than females. AS is characterized by obstruction of blood flow from the left ventricle to the aorta. In neonates, critical AS is almost always due to obstruction at the valve level. Associated congenital heart defects include left ventricular hypoplasia, mitral valve hypoplasia/stenosis, and coarctation of the aorta. A loud harsh systolic ejection murmur may be present. With critical stenosis of the aortic valve, the typical ejection click of aortic valve opening is often absent.

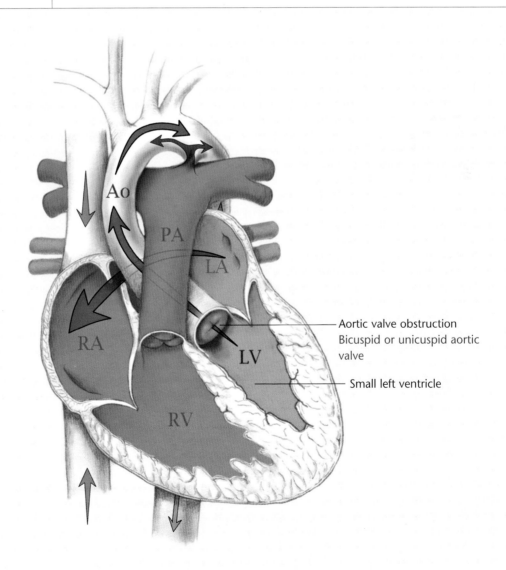

Aortic valve obstruction
Bicuspid or unicuspid aortic valve

Small left ventricle

Figure 2.47. Anatomic features of critical aortic valve stenosis.

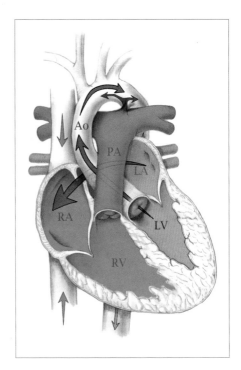

Figure 2.48. Critical aortic valve stenosis with a closing ductus arteriosus. Depending on the amount of valvular obstruction, a variable amount of blood will be ejected into the aorta. As the ductus closes, systemic and retrograde aortic blood flow (to the neck and coronary vessels), will diminish.

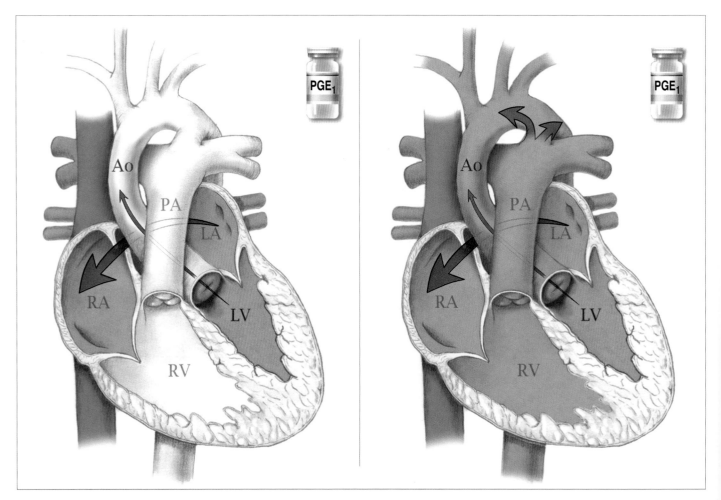

Figure 2.49. Pattern of blood flow seen when PGE₁ re-establishes ductal patency. Blood will shunt right-to-left from the pulmonary artery to the aorta and then systemic circulation. If aortic valve stenosis is severe, blood will also flow *retrograde* to the head, neck, and coronary vessels in order to perfuse these areas.

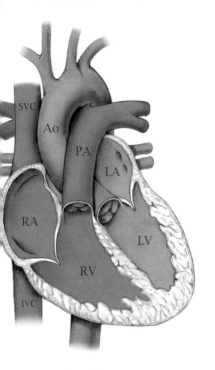

Normal heart

Interrupted Aortic Arch (IAA)

IAA accounts for approximately 1% of all cases of CHD and is characterized by complete discontinuity of the proximal and distal portions of the aortic arch. A right-to-left shunt through the PDA supplies all of the blood flow to the distal aorta. A VSD is frequently present and allows left-to-right shunting of oxygenated blood from the left ventricle to the pulmonary artery. There is a high association with 22q11 deletion syndrome.

Two types of IAA are most frequently observed:
- Type A involves interruption of the aorta distal to the left subclavian artery (LSCA).
- Type B is most common and involves interruption of the aorta between the left carotid artery and left subclavian artery (shown below).

Exam tip:

Type A: With ductal closure, the right and left brachial pulses would be equal, while femoral pulses would feel decreased.

Type B: With ductal closure, the left brachial pulse and femoral pulses would be decreased compared to the right brachial pulse.

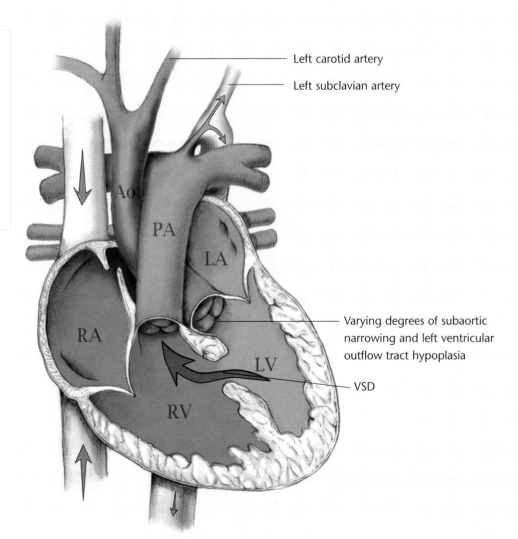

Figure 2.50. Anatomic features of IAA.

Left outflow tract CHD
Ductal dependent for SBF

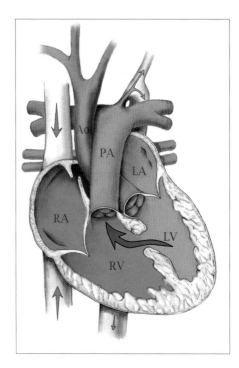

Figure 2.51. IAA with a closing ductus arteriosus. Depending on where the interruption occurs, blood flow to the area supplied by the right-to-left shunt through the ductus arteriosus will diminish, resulting in tissue hypoxia and shock.

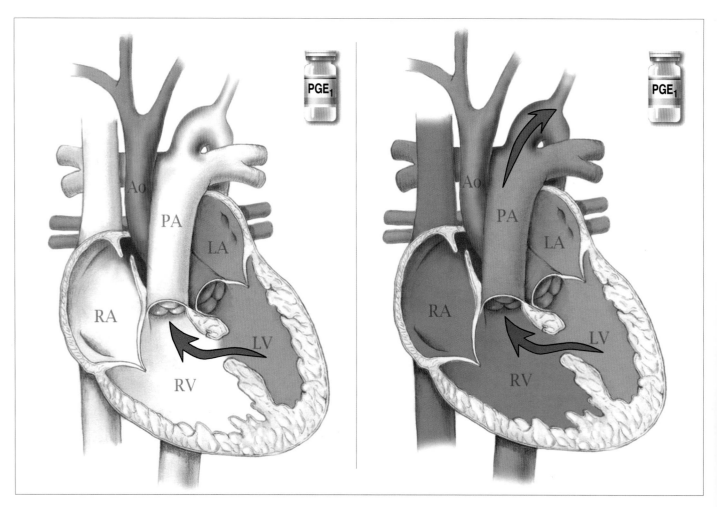

Figure 2.52. Pattern of blood flow seen when PGE₁ re-establishes ductal patency. Oxygenated blood will shunt from the left ventricle through the VSD to the pulmonary artery and then to the systemic circulation via a right-to-left ductal shunt.

Hypoplastic Left Heart Syndrome (HLHS)

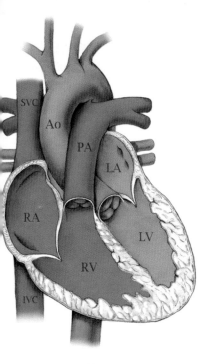

Normal heart

HLHS accounts for approximately 1% of all cases of CHD, and is characterized by the following:

- Hypoplasia of the left ventricle;
- Either severe mitral valve stenosis or atresia, or severe aortic valve stenosis or atresia; and
- Hypoplastic ascending aorta and transverse aortic arch.

Coarctation of the aorta is a frequent finding. It is important to realize that blood flow to *all regions* of the body is dependent on right-to-left ductal shunting (PA to aorta). To perfuse the brain, coronaries, head, and neck, blood must shunt from the PA through the ductus into the aorta, including *retrograde* in the ascending aorta. To perfuse the rest of the body, blood must shunt right to left *down* the descending aorta. As the ductus closes, perfusion is decreased to all organs, including the brain and heart.

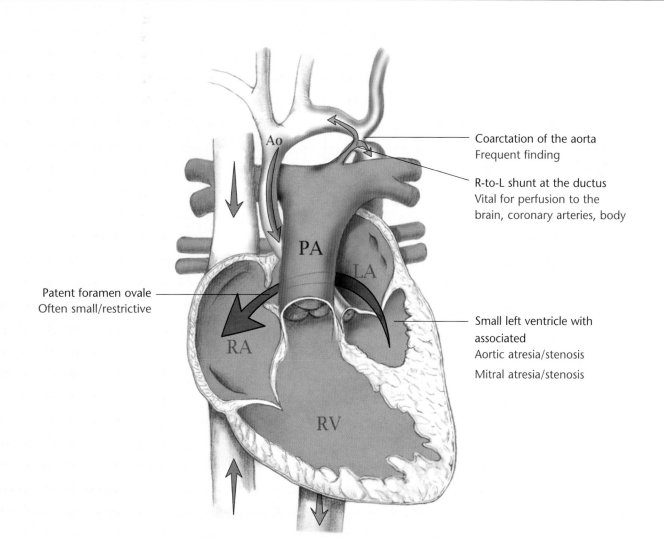

Coarctation of the aorta
Frequent finding

R-to-L shunt at the ductus
Vital for perfusion to the brain, coronary arteries, body

Patent foramen ovale
Often small/restrictive

Small left ventricle with associated
Aortic atresia/stenosis
Mitral atresia/stenosis

Figure 2.53. Anatomic features of HLHS.

Left outflow tract CHD
Ductal dependent for SBF

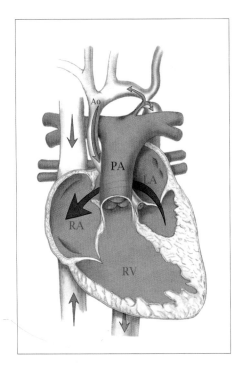

Hypoplastic Left Heart Syndrome (HLHS)

Figure 2.54. HLHS with a closing ductus arteriosus. As the ductus closes, the entire systemic circulation is compromised, resulting in severe shock.

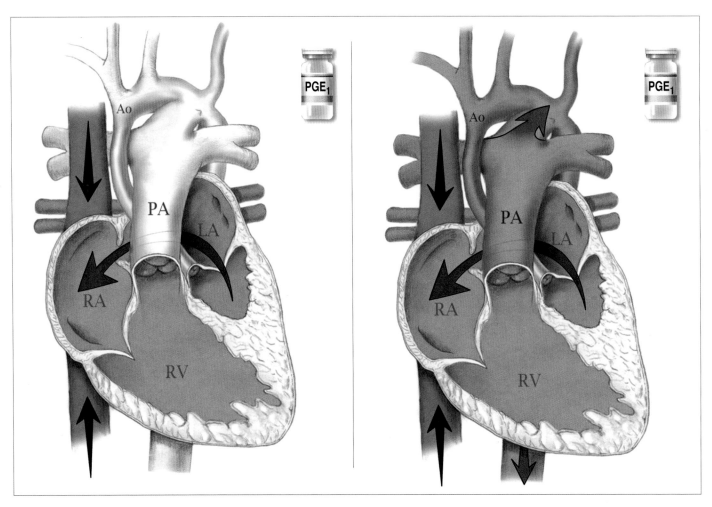

Figure 2.55. Pattern of blood flow seen when PGE₁ re-establishes ductal patency. Pulmonary venous return will shunt left to right to the right atrium. A variable amount of blood will then shunt right to left through the ductus arteriosus to perfuse the body, including the head, neck and coronary vessels.

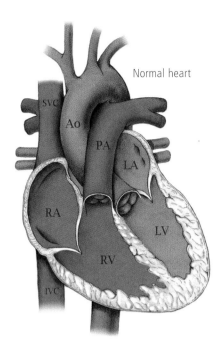

Normal heart

COA, AS, IAA, HLHS

Clinical Presentation

The clinical presentation for severe coarctation, critical aortic stenosis, interrupted aortic arch, and hypoplastic left heart syndrome, is similar, and often mimics severe sepsis with low cardiac output. As the ductus arteriosus begins to close, caregivers are likely to observe signs and symptoms of heart failure, including tachypnea, poor feeding, low urine output, differential blood pressures and a change in the level of consciousness. With further constriction of the ductus, a decrease in systemic perfusion leads to signs of shock: weak, thready pulses, prolonged capillary refill time, tachycardia, hypotension, dyspnea, and oliguria or anuria. Left untreated, most neonates with severe left heart obstruction will die.

Cyanosis

Differential cyanosis may be observed with right-to-left shunting through the ductus arteriosus.

Heart sounds

An ejection click may be present with aortic valve stenosis.

The second heart sound may be single.

With decreased ventricular function and heart failure, a gallop rhythm may be audible.

Murmur

Variable: In some cases, a systolic ejection murmur may be heard, while in other cases, no murmur is present.

Left outflow tract CHD
Ductal dependent for SBF

COA, AS, IAA, HLHS

Chest X-ray

Heart size

Cardiomegaly is the rule.

Pulmonary vasculature

Increased pulmonary vascular markings and evidence of pulmonary edema accompany the onset of congestive heart failure.

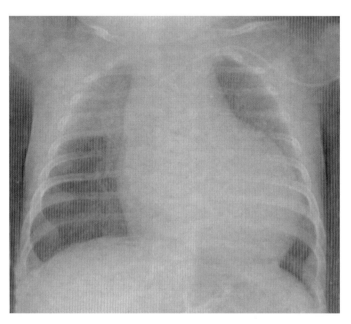

Figure 2.56. Neonate with COA. Right upper lobe atelectasis, pulmonary edema, and cardiomegaly are apparent. A central PICC line is in good position.

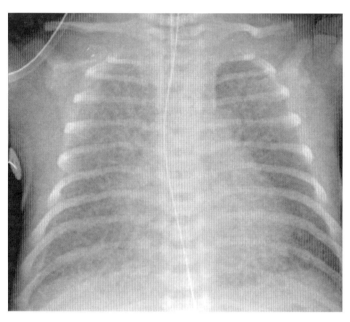

Figure 2.57. Neonate with AS. Cardiomegaly and congestive failure are evident. Note the interstitial and alveolar edema and small bilateral pleural effusions, R > L.

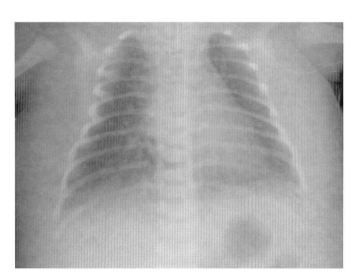

Figure 2.58. Neonate with IAA. Note the massive tissue and pulmonary edema. A central PICC line, ET tube, and gastric tube are all in good position.

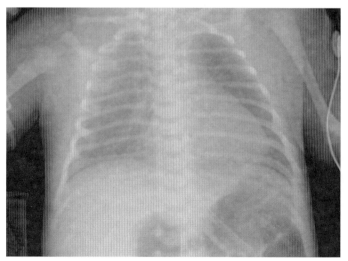

Figure 2.59. Neonate with HLHS. The baby is rotated making evaluation of heart size difficult. There is evidence of pulmonary congestion. A UAC is in good position at T7 and the ET tube is in good position in the mid-trachea. The OG tube tip is in the stomach.

COA, AS, IAA, HLHS

Initial Stabilization

Treatment is aimed at improving systemic blood flow, reversing metabolic acidosis, providing respiratory support, and assessing the degree of secondary organ damage suffered during the period of impaired organ perfusion.

1. Endotracheal intubation and mechanical ventilation are often required to reduce the work of breathing and strain on the heart.

2. An infusion of PGE_1 will help re-establish and maintain ductal patency and improve systemic perfusion. This usually relieves metabolic acidosis caused by tissue hypoxia.

3. Hyperoxia and hypocarbia should be avoided. Both decrease pulmonary vascular resistance, promoting increased pulmonary blood flow at the expense of right-to-left blood flow through the ductus arteriosus to the systemic circulation.

4. Ringer's lactate or normal saline volume support may be useful to improve systemic perfusion.

5. Inotropic support (dopamine, digoxin) may improve myocardial function.

6. Diuretics may be necessary to treat congestive heart failure.

7. Arm and leg blood pressures should be monitored frequently. Report differences (arm > leg) exceeding 15 mmHg.

8. NICU Management: Once the infant is stable, consult with cardiology or neonatology regarding the desired O_2 saturation range. O_2 saturation between 75 and 85% helps balance pulmonary blood flow (by increasing pulmonary vascular resistance) and systemic circulation (via the right-to-left ductal shunt). An elevated arterial PO_2 should be avoided because of its constrictive effects on ductal tissue and its vasodilatory effects on the pulmonary vasculature. If lung blood vessels dilate, more blood shunts to the lungs at the expense of the systemic circulation.

 Because of the right-to-left shunt at the ductus arteriosus, use extra caution with central venous catheters to prevent emboli from reaching the systemic circulation.

Left outflow tract CHD
Ductal dependent for SBF

S.T.A.B.L.E. Program

Introduction

Nurses and physicians involved with neonatal and emergency care will occasionally encounter neonates who are ill with cardiac conditions. Prompt, effective, and appropriate care can reduce secondary organ damage, improve short and long-term outcomes, and reduce morbidity and mortality. This section will discuss modifications to the six S.T.A.B.L.E. assessment components (**S**ugar, **T**emperature, **A**irway, **B**lood pressure, **L**ab work, and **E**motional support) necessary to care for neonates with suspected or confirmed CHD. For further information covered in the S.T.A.B.L.E. Program, the S.T.A.B.L.E. Learner manual is available at **www.stableprogram.org**.

Care must be provided based on the neonate's condition at presentation. If the baby is in shock, attention must first be devoted to reducing the work of breathing and identifying and treating primary causes of acid-base disturbances. Supportive and resuscitative measures include assisting ventilation and improving oxygenation, improving blood pressure and perfusion, establishing intravenous and arterial access, administering medications, and maintaining a normal body temperature.

General Guidelines

In the early phase of their illness, neonates challenged with the stress of cardiac disease usually do not tolerate enteral feedings. Significant respiratory distress, hypoxemia, or hypoxia can interfere with their ability to coordinate suck, swallow, and breathing. This increases the risk of aspiration during oral feedings and possibly during gavage feedings as well. Neonates affected by cardiac disease may also suffer intestinal ischemia during periods of poor systemic perfusion. With closure of the ductus arteriosus, in the presence of ductal dependent lesions, neonates will often display signs of increased distress, disinterest in feedings, a weak suck, and the development of intestinal ileus and vomiting. The safest approach is to withhold feedings and establish intravenous (IV) access as soon as possible. This will ensure that IV access is available for medications and fluid resuscitation needed emergently. In addition, placement of an IV will allow the infusion of appropriate glucose-containing solutions to support the increased energy demands of neonates with heart disease.

Glucose Production and Utilization Rate

In healthy term neonates, the steady-state glucose production/utilization rate is approximately 4 to 6 mg/kg/minute. Under stressful conditions or during illness, the glucose utilization rate may exceed the glucose production or availability rate, thus increasing the neonate's risk of developing hypoglycemia. Such stressful conditions include periods of anaerobic glycolysis, where glucose utilization is markedly accelerated, respiratory distress with labored breathing, septic and cardiogenic shock, and cold stress. Neonates with CHD may also suffer concurrent ailments that place them at higher risk for hypoglycemia. These include hyperinsulinemia, intrauterine growth restriction, the presence of chromosomal or genetic conditions, and prematurity.

Initial IV Fluid Rate and Infusion Guidelines

Once intravenous access is established, begin administering D10W at 80 ml/kg/day to provide a glucose infusion of 5.5 mg/kg/minute. In the absence of conditions related to hyperinsulinemia, neonates with limited or no glycogen stores (e.g., infants small for gestational age) or those with significantly increased glucose utilization, 5.5 mg/kg/minute is usually adequate to maintain the blood sugar above 50 mg/dL (2.8 mmol/L). The ideal target glucose level for sick neonates continues to be controversial. Nevertheless, 50 mg/dL (2.8 mmol/L) should ensure serum glucose levels recommended in current neonatal texts. Depending on the diagnosis, patient age, renal function, and laboratory values, the addition of electrolytes, calcium, and magnesium to the IV solution may be indicated. For guidance in this area, refer to neonatology resources or consult neonatal experts as needed.

A neonate who develops shock is at increased risk for acute renal failure, oliguria, and difficulty excreting adequate volumes of water. Hyponatremia, the appearance of edema, and development of congestive heart failure are associated with an imbalance between intake and output. If shock has occurred, and the patient is normoglycemic, consider decreasing the baseline fluid rate to 60 ml/kg/day (4.2 mg/kg/minute glucose infusion rate). It is often necessary to provide other fluids to expand the intravascular volume, often in the form of fluid boluses. Again, consultation with neonatal and cardiology experts is recommended as necessary.

Blood sugar levels should be monitored closely until a pattern of stability is established, and levels remain above 50 mg/dL. If the blood sugar is lower than desired, or the infant displays signs of hypoglycemia, the dextrose concentration may be increased to D12.5W or D15W. Details regarding glucose boluses may also be found in the S.T.A.B.L.E. Program learner manual or other neonatology texts. When glucose concentrations exceed D12.5W, it is customary to infuse fluids via a central venous line. Figures 3.1, 3.2, and the insert on page 105 offer guidance in the use of central catheters.

Intravenous Therapy

A minimum of two intravenous lines should be placed in neonates with suspected CHD. This will allow simultaneous infusion of medications (e.g., dopamine or PGE_1) and glucose-containing solutions. If possible, insert two peripheral IVs or an umbilical venous catheter (UVC) and a peripheral IV. A percutaneously inserted central catheter (PICC) may also be an excellent choice if skilled personnel can place and manage such a line.

All medications, including PGE_1, dopamine, and dobutamine may be infused via a peripheral IV or central venous catheter, as continuous drip infusions. PGE_1 is generally not compatible with any other medications, therefore, it should be infused by itself. PGE_1 should be infused through the most reliable line.

When using the UVC for medications and IV fluids, take extra care to ensure the catheter tip is properly positioned at the inferior vena cava/right atrial junction or just inside the right atrium (see Figure 3.1 for information regarding catheter location during emergency placement). When the radiographic appearance of the catheter displays the tip is in the mid-right atrium, the tip may actually have passed through the foramen ovale into the left atrium. All fluids or medications would then be infused directly into the systemic circulation, and this should be avoided.

Other benefits of umbilical venous catheters include the ability to monitor central venous pressure and, if cardiac catheterization is required, a route for accessing the heart. An umbilical arterial catheter (UAC) is indicated when continuous blood pressure monitoring and/or frequent arterial blood gas assessments are required. Dopamine and other vasopressors should never be given in an arterial line.

Umbilical catheter safety and general guidelines

1. Use sterile technique when placing lines, setting up infusions, drawing labs, and administering fluids. Do not advance a catheter into the baby once sterile technique has been disassembled.

2. Maintain an air-tight system. Do not allow air bubbles to infuse into the baby.

3. Check connections to be sure they are tight. Rapid, life-threatening blood loss can occur with inadvertent disconnection of the tubing.

4. Whenever possible, the UAC and UVC should be attached to a transducer. A dampened or flattened arterial waveform may indicate presence of an air bubble in the system, disconnection, development of thrombus in or around the catheter tip, hypotension, or changes in ductal patency.

5. If the catheter is repositioned, it is recommended that a chest or abdominal x-ray be repeated to confirm correct placement.

6. Monitor for complications related to an indwelling umbilical arterial catheter, in particular:

   a. Signs of arterial spasm, which include white, blue, or black discoloration of the skin in the back, buttocks, groin, legs, feet, or toes;

   b. The presence of a thrombus in or around the catheter tip, which may be observed by a dampened or flattened arterial waveform that may accompany changes in perfusion to the area below the thrombus;

   c. The development of hypertension or decreased urine output, which may reflect the occurrence of a renal artery embolus.

If any of the preceding signs are observed, they should be reported to the patient's practitioner or physician.

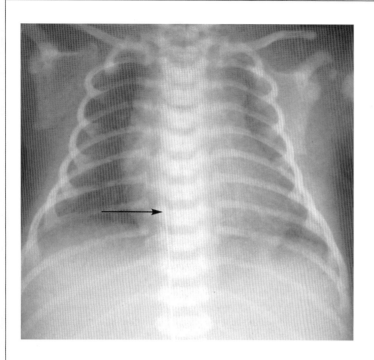

⚠ *Inadvertent overdose of heparin alters clotting and may cause severe hemorrhage. Double-check all heparin doses with another RN, physician, or pharmacist prior to administering this medication. The heparin vial may be confused with other similar vials. To avoid accidental overdose, discard the heparin vial after use.*

Figure 3.1. Umbilical venous catheters: guidelines for location, solutions, and medications.

Umbilical venous catheter (UVC)

Location

The catheter tip should be located above the diaphragm at the inferior vena cava (IVC)/right atrial (RA) junction. A tip located slightly in the right atrium is usually tolerated without complication. Insertion of the tip deep in the right atrium should be avoided because the tip may cross the foramen ovale to the left atrium.

Low position UVC – below the liver is appropriate only in an emergency

Under emergency conditions, a sterile umbilical catheter can be inserted 2 to 4 centimeters into the cord, until blood is freely obtained. The insertion depth is based on the baby's size. Remember that following birth and clamping of the umbilical cord there is no pulsatile flow in the umbilical vein. Therefore, all medications need to be flushed with several milliliters of sterile normal saline. If the tip is located near or in the liver, injury to liver tissue may result from infusion of hypertonic solutions.

IV fluid

- Continuous infusion of ≥ 1 ml per hour is usually adequate to keep the line patent.

- A 5 to 20% dextrose solution is appropriate if the tip is in good position.

- If a dextrose infusion is already being provided, some neonatologists prefer to infuse normal saline at 1 to 2 ml/hour to maintain central line patency.

- To avoid thrombus formation, heparin may be added to the IV fluid. The usual dose is 0.5 to 1 unit per ml of IV fluid.

Medications

If the tip is properly positioned above the diaphragm at the IVC/RA junction or just in the right atrium, a UVC can be used for most medications, including vasopressors.

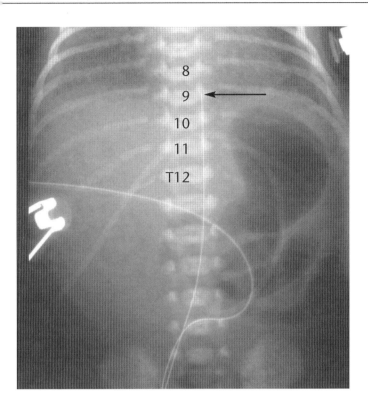

Figure 3.2. Umbilical arterial catheters: Guidelines for location, solutions, and medications.

Umbilical arterial catheter (UAC)

Location

High placement – the catheter tip should be located between T6 and T9.

Low placement – the catheter tip should be located between L3 and L4.

IV fluid

• Continuous infusion of ≥ 1 ml per hour is usually adequate to keep the line patent.

• A 5 to 15% dextrose solution is appropriate if the tip is in good position.

• If a dextrose infusion is already being provided, some neonatologists prefer to infuse normal saline at 1 to 2 ml/hour to maintain catheter patency.

• To avoid thrombus formation, heparin may be added to the IV fluid. The usual dose is 0.5 to 1 unit/ml of IV fluid.

Medications

A UAC is generally not recommended for administering medications.

 Never give vasopressors (e.g., dopamine, dobutamine, and epinephrine) in the UAC or any arterial line.

Neonates require constant thermal support to prevent the development of hypothermia. Consequences of severe hypothermia include stimulation of norepinephrine release, which causes pulmonary and peripheral vasoconstriction, the development of acidosis and hypoxemia, and even death. Babies who are born healthy receive routine care to prevent hypothermia: they are dried, wrapped in pre-warmed blankets, and held skin-to-skin by their mothers. Babies who are born ill, or who become ill, are vulnerable to hypothermia because normal routine care is altered.

For example, consider the five-day-old baby with ductal-dependent left-heart obstruction who develops shock when the ductus arteriosus begins to close. He is rushed to the hospital where he is undressed, examined, provided oxygen, and subjected to x-rays, lab draws, and the placement of IVs. During this dramatic resuscitation, his body temperature will drop and continue to drop until his caregivers turn their attention to reversing the decline.

Prevention is best! Caregivers often do not realize that infants experiencing hypoxia and anaerobic glycolysis are unable to effectively metabolize brown fat through chemical thermogenesis. Sick neonates are entirely dependent on their caregivers to maintain normal body temperatures. Do not fail to provide consistent thermal support.

Neonates with cardiac disease require varied levels of respiratory support, from saturation monitoring or oxygen supplementation to more intense therapies, including endotracheal intubation and assisted ventilation. Unless a neonate with CHD suffers concurrent respiratory illness known to diminish lung compliance, his or her lung compliance is usually normal or near normal. Therefore, conventional ventilator settings — positive inspiratory pressure (PIP), positive end-expiratory pressure (PEEP), inspiratory time (Ti), and rate (IMV) — are generally lower for neonates with cardiac disease than they are for neonates with respiratory disease. Hypocarbia and alkalemia may result from excessive ventilation, and overinflation of the lung may cause tissue injury and interfere with pulmonary blood flow. Take care to avoid these complications.

The Process of Oxygenation

Oxygen saturation is frequently monitored in the neonatal setting. Understanding the process of oxygen delivery and the oxygen-hemoglobin dissociation curve will help caregivers interpret the results obtained during monitoring. The process is therefore explained in the following paragraphs.

Figure 3.3 illustrates the process for cellular oxygen delivery. Oxygen diffuses from the alveoli through the interstitium of the lung into the pulmonary capillary blood, where it is bound by hemoglobin. The heart pumps red blood cells carrying oxygen through the arterial tree into the capillaries where oxygen diffusion from red cells to the tissues takes place to provide oxidative metabolism. The deoxygenated blood then returns to the heart and lungs for re-oxygenation.

Respiration $\rightarrow$ $\rightarrow$ $\rightarrow$ alveolar PO_2 rises $\rightarrow$ $\rightarrow$ $\rightarrow$ diffusion of O_2 through the interstitium of the lung $\rightarrow$ $\rightarrow$ $\rightarrow$ pulmonary capillaries $\rightarrow$ $\rightarrow$ $\rightarrow$ hemoglobin in RBCs binds O_2 $\rightarrow$ $\rightarrow$ $\rightarrow$ pumps hemoglobin and blood to tissues $\rightarrow$ $\rightarrow$ $\rightarrow$ hemoglobin releases O_2 $\rightarrow$ $\rightarrow$ $\rightarrow$ O_2 diffuses into tissues $\rightarrow$ $\rightarrow$ $\rightarrow$ O_2 diffuses through the cell membrane into the cells for normal cellular function.

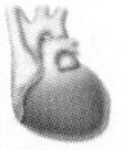

Figure 3.3. The process of cellular oxygen delivery.

Diffusion of oxygen from one point to the next occurs on a pressure gradient, from higher to lower: the PO_2 in arterial blood is higher than the PO_2 in tissue capillaries. This pressure gradient needs to be sufficient to allow for diffusion of oxygen from the lungs to the pulmonary capillary blood and again from the peripheral arterial blood to the tissue capillaries. Figure 3.4 illustrates the changes in PO_2 from 100 mmHg in the pulmonary alveolus, to 40 mmHg in the veins, to less than 30 mmHg in the tissues. It is interesting to note that the cells only require a PO_2 between 1 and 3 mmHg to carry out their normal chemical processes. Therefore, under conditions of near-complete lack of oxygen delivery to the cells, as seen with severe shock, ATP to maintain cell life may only be generated by anaerobic glycolysis. For very short periods of time, i.e., minutes, this type of metabolism will be sufficient to support cellular function. After that, failure to provide oxygen to the cells will result in death.

Alveolar PO_2 100 mmHg $\rightarrow$ $\rightarrow$ $\rightarrow$ venous capillary PO_2 40 mmHg $\rightarrow$ $\rightarrow$ $\rightarrow$ intracellular PO_2 averages 23 mmHg*.

* Under normal conditions, the cells require a PO_2 between 1 and 3 mmHg for normal cellular function.

Figure 3.4. Changes in average PO_2 from the alveolar space to the cell.

S.T.A.B.L.E. Program

109

Tissue hypoxia can result from many causes. Table 3.1 illustrates various factors that may interfere with oxygenation and oxygen delivery. These include pulmonary disease, which leads to failure to oxygenate pulmonary capillary blood; intracardiac mixing, which alters arterial PO_2; cardiac failure, which interferes with pumping of blood to the tissues and leads to pulmonary edema; anemia, which lowers O_2 content; and metabolic disorders at the cellular level such as an increased metabolic rate (increased O_2 consumption), as seen with hypothermia. As mentioned previously, cellular well-being depends on having sufficient oxygen to carry out cellular chemical processes. Thus, the pulmonary-cardiac-vascular system must be able to supply those minimal levels of oxygen and other substrates to sustain life.

Table 3.1. Factors Interfering with Oxygenation and Oxygen Delivery	
Factor	**Effect**
Lung disease	Hypoxemia or a low blood oxygen level, results from ventilation/perfusion (V/Q) mismatch or intrapulmonary shunting. The former occurs with conditions like persistent pulmonary hypertension of the newborn (PPHN), where the alveoli are ventilated but pulmonary perfusion is impaired; the latter occurs with conditions like atelectasis or pneumonia, where perfusion is normal but alveolar ventilation is impaired. Neonates with cardiac disease may have concurrent pulmonary disease.
Intracardiac shunt	Mixing of deoxygenated with oxygenated blood lowers the PO_2 of blood ejected into the aorta.
Cardiac failure	The systemic (usually left) ventricle cannot adequately pump the blood presented to it from the lungs, resulting in an increase in ventricular filling and pulmonary venous pressure, which pushes plasma into the interstitium of the lung, giving rise to pulmonary edema. This edema then increases the diffusion barrier for oxygenation (alveoli to red blood cells). In addition, failure to adequately pump red blood cells to the tissues leads to tissue hypoxia.
Hemoglobin	An inadequate hemoglobin level lowers oxygen content. Altered hemoglobin binding secondary to acid-base imbalances, hypo- or hyperthermia, and the type of hemoglobin (fetal or adult), all affect saturation at any given PO_2.
Increased metabolic rate	Increased utilization of oxygen at the cellular level is seen with an increased metabolic rate and with anaerobic glycolysis.

Oxygen saturation

Oxygen is transported to the tissues bound to hemoglobin. Oxygen saturation is the percentage of hemoglobin bound to oxygen. The oxygen-hemoglobin dissociation curve shown in Figure 3.5 rises rapidly from a starting point of zero for both PO_2 and percent O_2 saturation. When the saturation of fetal hemoglobin, which is the predominant hemoglobin in the neonate, reaches 50%, the PO_2 is 20 mmHg; at 75% saturation, the PO_2 is 30; at 95% saturation the PO_2 is 70; and at 98%, the PO_2 is 100. If alveolar oxygenation is high, which may occur when the infant is breathing supplemental oxygen, the saturation will change by only one or two percent, to a maximum of 100%, but the amount of dissolved oxygen will increase substantially such that the PO_2 may reach 300 or 400 mmHg.

Shift to the left or shift to the right

A shift in the oxygen-hemoglobin dissociation curve to the left or right affects the saturation at any given PO_2 level and affects the ability of hemoglobin to release oxygen to the tissues. When the curve is shifted to the left, as in the presence of fetal hemoglobin, alkalemia, hypocarbia, and hypothermia, the saturation will be higher for any given PO_2, but the hemoglobin will less readily release oxygen to the tissues. When the curve is shifted to the right, as seen with acidemia, hypercarbia, and hyperthermia, the saturation will be lower for any given PO_2, but the hemoglobin will more readily release oxygen to the tissues.

Saturation, Hemoglobin, and CHD

Parents and caregivers frequently ask how an infant with cyanotic congenital heart disease tolerates an O_2 saturation between 75 and 85%. The answer lies in the ability of hemoglobin to release adequate amounts of oxygen to the tissues. This ability, however, depends on the infant's condition, including cardiac output, tissue perfusion, type and amount of hemoglobin, pH, and body temperature.

To ensure that adequate amounts of hemoglobin are available to carry oxygen, optimizing the hemoglobin and hematocrit may warrant transfusion of packed red blood cells. The target hemoglobin level is individualized based on the patient's condition, underlying cardiac anomaly, and the degree of cyanosis.

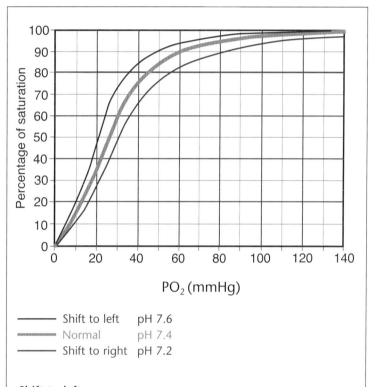

Shift to left   pH 7.6
Normal   pH 7.4
Shift to right   pH 7.2

Shift-to-left curve:
1. Fetal hemoglobin
2. Decreased hydrogen ions (higher pH)
3. Decreased CO_2
4. Decreased temperature

Shift-to-right curve:
1. Increased hydrogen ions (lower pH)
2. Increased CO_2
3. Increased temperature
4. Increased 2,3-diphosphoglycerate (DPG)

Figure 3.5. Oxygen-hemoglobin dissociation curve.

S.T.A.B.L.E. Program

Oxygen content

At 37° Celsius, one gram of hemoglobin binds 1.34 mls of oxygen as shown in Figure 3.6. Under normal conditions, a negligible amount of oxygen is also dissolved in plasma and is not included in the calculation of oxygen content. When the hemoglobin is 20 gm/dL, the oxygen content in 100 ml of whole blood is approximately 27 ml. When the hemoglobin is 10 gm/dL, the oxygen content for the same volume of blood is only 13.4 ml. For support of metabolism, the tissues require approximately 5 mls of oxygen for every 100 mls of blood perfusing them.

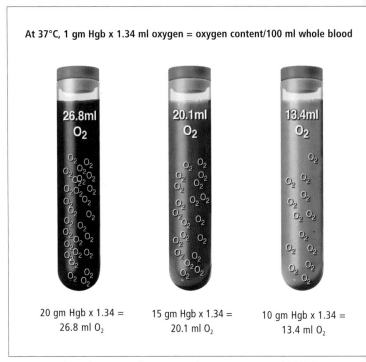

At 37°C, 1 gm Hgb x 1.34 ml oxygen = oxygen content/100 ml whole blood

26.8ml O_2

20.1ml O_2

13.4ml O_2

20 gm Hgb x 1.34 = 26.8 ml O_2

15 gm Hgb x 1.34 = 20.1 ml O_2

10 gm Hgb x 1.34 = 13.4 ml O_2

Figure 3.6. Effect of varying hemoglobin levels on oxygen content.

Cyanosis

The color of reduced hemoglobin, or hemoglobin that is not bound to oxygen, is purple. It takes at least 3 to 5 grams/dL of reduced hemoglobin for cyanosis to be apparent. This has implications for both low and high hemoglobin levels. Figure 3.7 illustrates these concepts.

A neonate with a normal hemoglobin level (15 gm/dL) will appear cyanotic when O₂ saturation declines to around 80%. To understand this calculation and therefore be able to predict when cyanosis will be apparent for any baseline hemoglobin value, take 3 grams of hemoglobin, (which is the minimum amount of desaturated hemoglobin needed for clinical cyanosis), and divide by the total hemoglobin value of 15 gm/dL. The result is 0.2 or 20%; so 100% (saturated hemoglobin) minus 20% (desaturated hemoglobin) results in 80% saturation. Remember, when the saturation is 85% or 90%, some reduced hemoglobin is already circulating. With desaturation of only 1 to 2 more grams/dL of hemoglobin, cyanosis may become apparent.

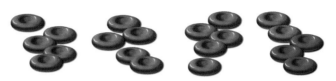

Hgb 20 gm/dL — O₂ saturation 85% and cyanosis is apparent

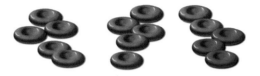

Hgb 15 gm/dL — O₂ saturation 80% and cyanosis is apparent

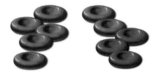

Hgb 10 gm/dL — O₂ saturation 70% and cyanosis is apparent

Red RBCs represent 1 gram of saturated hemoglobin

Purple RBCs represent 1 gram of desaturated hemoglobin

Figure 3.7. Hemoglobin, oxygen saturation, and cyanosis. In the presence of polycythemia (hemoglobin ≥ 20 gm/dL or a venous hematocrit of approximately 65%), desaturation of 3 grams/dL of fetal hemoglobin results in a PO₂ of 40 and an O₂ saturation of 85%, (example pertains to desaturation of a hemoglobin value of 20 gm/dL). Providing tissue perfusion is normal, tissue hypoxia will not result because oxygen content is good. With anemia (hemoglobin ≤ 10 gm/dL), however, cyanosis may not be apparent until more than 30–50% (3 to 5 gm/dL) of the hemoglobin is reduced (not carrying oxygen). When the hemoglobin is 10 gm/dL, desaturation of 3 to 5 gm/dL will result in a PO₂ between 20 and 28 mmHg. The oxygen content would also be lower, thus increasing the risk for tissue hypoxia.

Procedures for Assessing Oxygenation and Saturation

Hyperoxia test (100% O_2 challenge test or shunt study)

Information obtained from this procedure may be useful for differentiating cardiac from pulmonary disease.

1. While the infant is breathing room air, obtain a right radial (pre-ductal) arterial blood gas. This is an optional step if the patient is cyanotic on room air.

2. Place the infant on 100% oxygen via a hood.

3. After 10 to 15 minutes, repeat or obtain a right radial arterial blood gas.

4. If the PO_2 obtained on 100% oxygen rises above 150 mmHg, significant intracardiac shunting secondary to cyanotic CHD is unlikely and pulmonary causes of hypoxemia become more likely.

 An infant with severe, life-threatening, ductal-dependent left heart obstructive CHD may have a $PO_2 > 150$ mmHg.

In addition, relying on changes in oxygen saturation alone may misguide interpretation. Obtaining arterial blood gases in the manner just described is recommended for an accurate evaluation.

Evaluation of pre-and post-ductal saturation or PO_2

Indications

To detect right-to-left shunting at the ductus arteriosus.

Equipment

For this procedure, you will need two pulse oximeters or, if two monitors are not available, you can place the probe on the right hand for several minutes, and then move the probe to the foot for several minutes. Record and compare the O_2 saturation in the right hand and either foot.

1. Place an oximeter probe on the right hand and either foot.

2. To evaluate arterial PO_2 instead of saturation, obtain an arterial blood gas from the right radial artery (pre-ductal) and from the umbilical artery or posterior tibialis artery (post-ductal).

3. If there is a right-to-left shunt at the ductus arteriosus, the O_2 saturation (or PO_2) in the right hand or wrist will be higher than the O_2 saturation (or PO_2) in areas served by the distal aorta (legs or umbilical artery).

4. The exception is seen with transposition of the great arteries, in which case the pre-ductal (right hand) saturation may be lower than the post-ductal (leg saturation). This is known as *reverse differential cyanosis.*

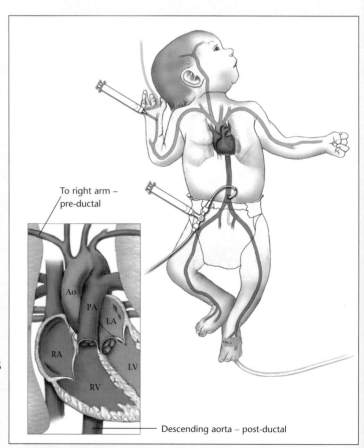

To right arm – pre-ductal

Ao
PA
LA
RA
LV
RV

Descending aorta – post-ductal

Figure 3.8. Illustration of pre- and post- ductal saturation patterns when there is a right-to-left shunt at the ductus arteriosus.

Cardiac output

Cardiac output is influenced by heart rate and stroke volume (heart rate multiplied by stroke volume equals cardiac output). The neonatal myocardium however, is poorly compliant and has limited capacity to increase stroke volume. Therefore, in order to increase cardiac output, the neonatal heart rate increases, resulting in tachycardia.

In addition to electrolyte, mineral, or energy imbalances, factors that negatively affect cardiac output include a decrease in preload (volume of venous return), an increase in afterload or vascular resistance (myocardial work increases as resistance increases), or decreased myocardial contractility. Abnormalities in any of these areas may result in varying degrees of decompensation. If these abnormalities are untreated and persistent, the neonate may deteriorate and become critically ill.

Shock

A neonate with severe congenital heart disease, poor cardiac output, and/or severe hypoxemia is at risk for developing shock. Delayed or insufficient treatment may lead to permanent tissue injury, organ damage, and death. Rapid, effective treatment of shock may include respiratory support to increase tissue oxygenation and decrease work of breathing, volume resuscitation to increase preload and cardiac output, identification and treatment of primary causes of acid-base disturbances, and medications and therapies to improve heart function (inotropy).

Because hypotension is a late sign of cardiac decompensation, blood pressure may be normal when in fact the neonate is experiencing the early stages of shock. Identification and treatment of shock must be based on the history, physical exam, and laboratory assessment, not on an isolated blood pressure measurement.

Blood and pulse pressure

Figure 3.9 demonstrates graphs of normal arterial blood pressure values in neonates of varying weights. To use these graphs, you must first determine the baby's weight in kilograms. Measure the blood pressure and then plot the systolic, diastolic, and mean values on each of the corresponding graphs. The area within the solid lines is considered normal.

Determine the pulse pressure by subtracting the diastolic from the systolic measurement. A normal pulse pressure in a term neonate is between 25 and 30 mmHg and in a preterm infant between 15 and 25 mmHg. A narrow pulse pressure may indicate peripheral vasoconstriction, heart failure, or low cardiac output. A wide pulse pressure may indicate a large aortic runoff, as seen with a significant patent ductus arteriosus or large arteriovenous malformation.

Blood transfusion

If a blood transfusion is necessary, packed red blood cells should be irradiated, washed, and filtered. Some pediatric cardiologists recommend cytomegalovirus (CMV) negative blood. This becomes particularly important in the infant with hypoplastic left heart syndrome who is being considered for a heart transplant. Usually, 10 to 15 ml/kg of packed red blood cells are transfused, the amount dependent upon the desired hemoglobin. Consultation with a pediatric cardiologist, neonatologist, or nurse practitioner will help identify cardiac patients who may benefit from transfusion therapy to maximize oxygen carrying capacity.

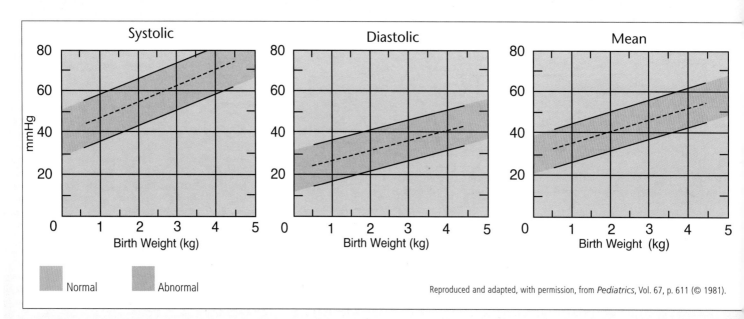

Normal   Abnormal

Reproduced and adapted, with permission, from *Pediatrics*, Vol. 67, p. 611 (© 1981).

Figure 3.9. Normal blood pressure values in well newborns of varying weights.

Initial studies to evaluate the condition of neonates with suspected or confirmed congenital heart disease may include the following tests. The inclusion or exclusion of tests is dictated by the patient's history and condition.

1. **Blood gas.** Arterial sampling allows for assessment of oxygenation, ability to remove carbon dioxide, and acid-base status. Capillary samples are useful for evaluating CO_2 removal and acid-base status, but are not useful for evaluating oxygenation.

2. **Complete blood count with differential (CBC with diff).** This test allows for the assessment of anemia, polycythemia, and thrombocytopenia. In addition, clinicians consider both the white blood cell count and differential when evaluating the infant for infection. Remember, however, that some neonates suffering from infection have a normal white blood cell count and/or differential. Therefore, the decision to treat infection must be based on a careful consideration of the history, clinical presentation, and physical examination, rather than an isolated CBC result.

3. **Blood sugar (serum glucose).** As discussed in the Sugar section, neonates with CHD are at increased risk for hypoglycemia. Serum glucose values in neonates fluctuate based on stressors experienced during the course of illness. Be vigilant for signs and symptoms of hypoglycemia, which may be subtle, nonspecific, and commonly observed with other diseases, including CHD. These include cardiorespiratory findings — tachypnea, cyanosis, and apnea; and neurologic signs — tremors, jitteriness, irritability, abnormal or weak cry, disinterest in feeding or weak suck, lethargy, hypotonia, hypothermia, and in severe cases, seizures.

4. **Electrolytes, BUN, and creatinine.** These tests are useful for evaluating renal function, especially if the infant has experienced circulatory compromise, and to detect aberrations that may negatively affect heart function, including hypo- or hyperkalemia and hyponatremia, regardless of the underlying etiology.

5. **Calcium.** Low values may negatively affect myocardial contractility and require calcium supplementation. Patients with 22q11 deletion syndrome may have severe persistent hypocalcemia.

6. **Coagulation studies.** Prothrombin time (PT), partial thromboplastin time (PTT), and fibrinogen should be assessed if bleeding is observed or if there is a history of shock.

7. **Liver function tests.** These will help determine the degree of liver damage suffered during periods of shock or hepatic damage from other etiologies.

8. **Chromosomal analysis.** This test should be performed if physical features or history are suspicious for genetic or chromosomal abnormalities.

9. **FISH chromosomal analysis for 22q11 deletion.** If DiGeorge syndrome is suspected, this test provides definitive diagnosis (see page 19). A primary immunodeficiency panel to evaluate for an absent or hypoplastic thymus is also indicated. 22q11 deletion syndrome should be considered when the diagnosis includes any of the following types of CHD: interrupted aortic arch type B, truncus arteriosus, pulmonary atresia with ventricular septal defect, right aortic arch, abnormal origins of the branch pulmonary arteries, and tetralogy of Fallot.

S.T.A.B.L.E. Program

Imagine the shock when parents hear the words "we think there may be something wrong with your baby's heart." How absolutely frightening those words must sound. Parents must struggle to absorb their baby's complicated medical situation, one that frequently arrives without warning.

During the stabilization process, healthcare providers strive to provide timely, appropriate, and correctly performed care in order to optimize the outcome for the baby. Throughout this process, it is imperative that caregivers remain vigilant to the needs and concerns, spoken and unspoken, of the family.

The birth of a baby is considered a "life crisis," even in the best of circumstances. The birth of a sick baby creates immense stress and a different kind of crisis. This is a very disruptive time for the family. They will worry not only about their immediate situation, but also about the future. Will my child be "normal"? Will he or she be able to play like other children? Will he or she endure pain? Will he or she be scarred? Will he or she be able to learn? What will this mean for our family, our lifestyle, and our other children? Parents may not come right out and voice these concerns during the period when you interface with them, but these concerns are naturally there.

Healthcare providers are in an ideal position to influence adaptation to this crisis. It is important to recognize sources of parental stress in the neonatal intensive care unit. These include "preexisting and concurrent personal and family factors, prenatal and perinatal experiences, infant illness, treatments and appearance, concerns about the infant's outcome, loss of the parental role, and health care providers" (Merenstein & Gardner, 2002, p. 730).

In their interactions with families, healthcare providers must balance appropriate display of sensitivity, flexibility, education, attitudes, and NICU policy. Today, many NICUs have adopted a model of family-centered neonatal care. This model maximizes collaboration among parents and professionals, allows the learning of parenting skills, and optimizes development of a healthy parent-child relationship. Finally, healthcare providers must realize the importance of providing understandable, accurate educational tools so that parents may fully comprehend their child's medical issues.

Useful Resources for Healthcare Professionals and Parents

Cardiology

www.acc.org

This is the Web site of the American College of Cardiology's Congenital Heart Disease and Pediatric Cardiology Committee. The site is oriented to the professional. CHD-related news, information about grants and ongoing trials, standards, meetings, and educational materials may be found on this site.

www.americanheart.org

This is the Web site of the American Heart Association. Click on Site Index, then Children: Heart Disease & Health where you will find a wealth of information for parents and professionals.

Genetics

The following Web sites offer information on genetic problems and risks.

http://www.marchofdimes.com/gyponline/index.bm2

This section of the March of Dimes Web site offers the "Genetics & Your Practice Curriculum," which consists of a 190-page resource guide to help primary care and social service professionals:

• Evaluate patients at risk for developing genetic disorders;

• Identify patients who may benefit from genetic services;

• Access referral, testing, diagnosis, and interventions for affected patients; and

• Address financial, ethical, legal and social issues.

www.ndss.org

The National Down Syndrome Society Web site is a comprehensive source of information on Down syndrome.

www.trisomy.org

This is the Web site of the Support Organization for Trisomy 18, 13, and Related Disorders (S.O.F.T.), a nonprofit volunteer organization offering support for parents who have had a child with a chromosome disorder, and education to families and professionals interested in the care of these children.

March of Dimes Nursing Modules

These nursing modules are designed to help perinatal nurses integrate scientific and clinical advances into the care of mothers and babies. For more information, please visit the March of Dimes Web site:

www.marchofdimes.com/nursing

To order modules, call the March of Dimes Fulfillment Center (800) 367-6630 or (770) 280-4115.

Breastfeeding the Infant with Special Needs, 2nd Edition (2007)
Donna Dowling, PhD, RN
Gail McCain, PhD, RN, FAAN

Provides evidence-based practice guidelines to promote successful breastfeeding for infants with special needs, including preterm infants and infants with cleft lip and palate, congenital heart disease, Down syndrome and hypotonia. Emphasizes the nurse's role in facilitating successful breastfeeding for these infants. Recommends resources for parents and health care professionals. Item #33-1994-05.

Cultural Competence in the Care of Childbearing Families (2003)
Mary Lou Moore, PhD, RNC, FACCE, FAAN
Merry-K. Moos, BSN, FNP, MPH

Provides information on culturally competent nursing care of childbearing women and their families, including U.S. demographics; cultural perspectives, traditions, and characteristics; nutrition and physiologic differences; cultural assessment; and ethical issues. Also presents profiles of 13 different cultural groups with information on prenatal care, labor and birth, and postpartum care. Item #33-1656-02.

Discharge and Follow-Up of the High-Risk Preterm Infant (2001)
Susan Bakewell-Sachs, PhD, RN, CS-CPNP
Susan Blackburn, PhD, RN, C, FAAN

Presents information on discharge management, transition to home, and post-discharge issues for preterm infants and their families. Focuses on recovering preterm infants who are discharged on medications but who are otherwise not dependent upon technological support. Item #33-1433-00.

Useful Resources for Healthcare Professionals and Parents

Embryonic and Fetal Evaluation During Pregnancy (2002)
Marilyn Stringer, PhD, CRNP, RDMS
Barrie Essner, MSN, CRNP

Provides a broad understanding of intrauterine surveillance, including growth, development, and teratogenic agents; genetic screening; ultrasound evaluation; and fetal well-being studies. Item #33-1520-01.

Genetic Issues for Perinatal Nurses, 2nd Edition (2003)
Janet K. Williams, PhD, RN, CPNP, CGC, FAAN
Dale Halsey Lea, MPH, RN, APNG[c], FAAN

Includes an update of genetic discoveries for inherited diseases and birth defects and discussion of genetics-related ethical issues and nursing responsibilities for reproducing families. Addresses collection, recording, and interpretation of genetic information; genetic resources and referrals; informed consent; and management of individuals with genetic conditions. Item #33-1751-02.

Loss and Grieving in Pregnancy and the First Year of Life: A Caring Resource for Nurses (2002)
Penelope Buschman Gemma, MS, RN, CS, FAAN
Joan Arnold, PhD, RN

Discusses grief associated with death during the perinatal through postnatal periods; heightens nursing awareness and understanding of parental and family grief; and describes nursing interventions and support mechanisms for working with grieving families. Item #33-1547-01.

Preterm Labor: Prevention and Nursing Management, 3rd Edition (2004)
Margaret Comerford Freda, EdD, RN, CHES, FAAN
Ellen Tate Patterson, DSN, RN

Presents pathophysiology of preterm labor, diagnostic criteria, history of preterm birth prevention programs, and preterm labor prevention strategies. Discusses nursing management of women hospitalized with preterm labor, women being treated for preterm labor in the home and women facing inevitable preterm delivery. Item # 33-1805-03.

Sexually Transmitted Infections, Including HIV: Impact on Women's Reproductive Health (2008)
Catherine Ingram Fogel, PhD, RN, FAAN
Beth Perry Black, MSN, BSN

Provides clinical information about sexually transmitted infections (STIs). Includes information on the scope of the problem, pathogens, epidemiology, risk factors, transmission, and complications. Identifies nursing interventions for women's sexual health, safer sex guidelines, screening, and counseling. Addresses treatment guidelines from the Centers for Disease Control and Prevention (CDC). Item # 33-2082-06.

The Premature Infant: Nursing Assessment and Management, 2nd Edition (2007)
Lyn E. Vargo, PhD, NNP, RNC
Carol Wiltgen Trotter, PhD, NNP, RNC

Focuses on the most common physiologic problems seen in premature infants after birth. Addresses incidence, pathophysiology, respiratory distress syndrome, bronchopulmonary dysplasia, apnea of prematurity, patent ductus arteriosus, retinopathy of prematurity, neonatal sepsis, meningitis, pneumonia, necrotizing enterocolitis, and intraventricular hemorrhage. Item # 33-1995-05.

Tobacco, Alcohol and Drug Use in Childbearing Families (2008)
Margaret H. Kearney, PhD, RN, FAAN

Provides an overview of the extent and impact of tobacco, alcohol and other drug use by pregnant women in the United States. Gives nurses evidence-based strategies to support families dealing with these issues. Presents current knowledge about the effects of commonly used substances on maternal and child health. Describes nursing strategies for assessment, intervention and referral. Discusses social and ethical issues. Item # 33-2196-07.

References

Allen, H.D., Phillips, J.R. & Chan, D.P. (2001). History and physical examination. In H.D. Allen, H.P. Gutgesell, E.B. Clark & D.J. Driscoll (Eds.), *Moss and Adams' heart disease in infants, children, and adolescents* (6th ed., pp. 143–152). Philadelphia: Lippincott Williams & Wilkins.

Ammari, A.N. & Schulze, K.F. (2002). Uses and abuses of sodium bicarbonate in the neonatal intensive care unit. *Current Opinions in Pediatrics*, 14, 151-156.

Barber, G. (1998). Hypoplastic left heart syndrome. In A. Garson, Jr., J. T. Bricker, D.J. Fisher & S.R. Neish (Eds.), *The science and practice of pediatric cardiology* (2nd ed., pp. 1625–1645). Baltimore: Williams & Wilkins.

Beekman, R.H, III. (2001). Coarctation of the aorta. In H.D. Allen, H.P. Gutgesell, E.B. Clark & D.J. Driscoll (Eds.), *Moss and Adams' heart disease in infants, children, and adolescents* (6th ed., pp. 988–1010). Philadelphia: Lippincott Williams & Wilkins.

Bengur, A.R. (1998). Truncus arteriosus. In A. Garson, Jr., J. T. Bricker, D.J. Fisher & S.R. Neish (Eds.), *The science and practice of pediatric cardiology* (2nd ed., pp. 1421–1430). Baltimore: Williams & Wilkins.

Chameides, L., & Hazinski, M.F. (Eds.). (1999). Pediatric advanced life support, 1997– 99: *Emergency cardiovascular care programs*. (pp. 9.7–9.8). Dallas, TX: American Heart Association.

Corbet, A.J. (1998). Medical manipulation of the ductus arteriosus. In A. Garson, Jr., J. T. Bricker, D.J. Fisher & S.R. Neish (Eds.), *The science and practice of pediatric cardiology* (2nd ed., pp. 2489–2513). Baltimore: Williams & Wilkins.

Cornelli, H.M. (1993). Evaluation, treatment, and transport of pediatric patents with shock. *Pediatric Clinics of North America, 40* (2), 303–319.

Craig, J.E., Scholz, T.A., Vanderhooft, S.L., & Etheridge, S.P. (1998). Fat necrosis after ice application for supraventricular tachycardia termination. *Journal of Pediatrics*, 133 (6), 727.

Danford, D.A. & McNamara, D.G. (1998). Infants with congenital heart disease in the first year of life. In A. Garson, Jr., J. T. Bricker, D.J. Fisher & S.R. Neish (Eds.), *The science and practice of pediatric cardiology* (2nd ed., pp. 2227–2241). Baltimore: Williams & Wilkins.

Danford, D.A. & McNamara, D.G. (1998). Innocent murmurs and heart sounds. In A. Garson, Jr., J. T. Bricker, D.J. Fisher & S.R. Neish (Eds.), *The science and practice of pediatric cardiology* (2nd ed., pp. 2203–2212). Baltimore: Williams & Wilkins.

Driscoll, D.J. (1998). Tricuspid atresia. In A. Garson, Jr., J. T. Bricker, D.J. Fisher & S.R. Neish (Eds.), *The science and practice of pediatric cardiology* (2nd ed., pp. 1579–1587). Baltimore: Williams & Wilkins.

Driscoll, D.J. (1999). Left-to-right shunt lesions. *Pediatric Clinics of North America*, 46 (2), 355–368.

Duff, D.F. & McNamara, D.G. (1998). History and physical examination of the cardiovascular system. In A. Garson, Jr., J. T. Bricker, D.J. Fisher & S.R. Neish (Eds.), *The science and practice of pediatric cardiology* (2nd ed., pp. 693–713). Baltimore: Williams & Wilkins.

Earing, M., Ackerman, M.J. & Driscoll, D.J. (2002). Cardiac phenotype in the chromosome 22 q11.2 microdeletion syndrome. *Progress in Pediatric Cardiology*. 15, 119–123.

Epstein, M.L. (2001). Congenital stenosis and insufficiency of the tricuspid valve. In H.D. Allen, H.P. Gutgesell, E.B. Clark & D.J. Driscoll (Eds.), *Moss and Adams' heart disease in infants, children, and adolescents* (6th ed., pp. 810–819). Philadelphia: Lippincott Williams & Wilkins.

Epstein, M.L. (2001). Tricuspid atresia. In H.D. Allen, H.P. Gutgesell, E.B. Clark & D.J. Driscoll (Eds.), *Moss and Adams' heart disease in infants, children, and adolescents* (6th ed., pp. 799–809). Philadelphia: Lippincott Williams & Wilkins.

Fedderly, R.T. (1999). Left ventricular outflow obstruction. *Pediatric Clinics of North America, 46* (2), 369–384.

Fiser, D.H. (1997). Intraosseous infusions. In R.A. Dieckmann, D.H. Fiser, & S.M. Selbst (Eds.), *Illustrated textbook of pediatric emergency and critical care procedures* (pp. 220–224). St. Louis: Mosby.

Flanagan, M.F., Yeager, S.B., & Weindling, S.N. (1999). Cardiac disease. In G.B. Avery, M.A. Fletcher, & M.G. MacDonald (Eds.), Neonatology: *Pathophysiology and management of the newborn* (pp. 577–646). Philadelphia: Lippincott Williams & Wilkins.

Freed, M.D. (2001). Aortic stenosis. In H.D. Allen, H.P. Gutgesell, E.B. Clark & D.J. Driscoll (Eds.), *Moss and Adams' heart disease in infants, children, and adolescents* (6th ed., pp. 970–987). Philadelphia: Lippincott Williams & Wilkins.

Freedom, R.M., Black, M.D. & Benson, L.N. (2001). Hypoplastic left heart syndrome. In H.D. Allen, H.P. Gutgesell, E.B. Clark & D.J. Driscoll (Eds.), *Moss and Adams' heart disease in infants, children, and adolescents* (6th ed., pp. 1011–1026). Philadelphia: Lippincott Williams & Wilkins.

Freedom, R.M. & Nykanen, D.G. (2001). Pulmonary atresia and intact ventricular septum. In H.D. Allen, H.P. Gutgesell, E.B. Clark & D.J. Driscoll (Eds.), *Moss and Adams' heart disease in infants, children, and adolescents* (6th ed., pp. 845–863). Philadelphia: Lippincott Williams & Wilkins.

Gardner, S.L., Johnson, J.L., & Lubchenco, L.O. (2002). Initial nursery care. In G.B. Merenstein & S.L. Gardner (Eds.), *Handbook of neonatal intensive care* (5th ed., pp. 725–753). St. Louis: Mosby.

References

Geva, T. & Van Praagh, S. (2001). Anomalies of the pulmonary veins. In H.D. Allen, H.P. Gutgesell, E.B. Clark & D.J. Driscoll (Eds.), *Moss and Adams' heart disease in infants, children, and adolescents* (6th ed., pp. 736–772). Philadelphia: Lippincott Williams & Wilkins.

Gewitz, M.H. (2001). Cardiac disease in the newborn infant. In R.A. Polin, M.C. Yoder & F.D. Burg (Eds.), *Workbook in practical neonatology* (3rd ed., pp. 251–298). Philadelphia: W.B. Saunders.

Glass, S.M. (1999). Routine care. In P.J. Thureen, J. Deacon, P. O'Neill, & J. Hernandez (Eds.), *Assessment and care of the well newborn* (pp. 188–193). Philadelphia: W.B. Saunders.

Grifka, R.G. (1999). Cyanotic congenital heart disease with increased pulmonary blood flow. *Pediatric Clinics of North America, 46* (2), 405–425.

Gutgesell, H.P. (1998). Cardiac malposition and heterotaxy. In A. Garson, Jr., J. T. Bricker, D.J. Fisher & S.R. Neish (Eds.), *The science and practice of pediatric cardiology* (2nd ed., pp. 1539–1561). Baltimore: Williams & Wilkins.

Guyton, A.C. & Hall, J.E. (Eds.). (2000). *Textbook of medical physiology* (10th ed., pp. 463–473). Philadelphia: W.B. Saunders.

Hannon, D.W. & Fairbrother, D.L. (2003). Arrhythmias and cardiac pacing. In R.M. Perkin, J.D. Swift, & D.A. Newton (Eds.), *Pediatric hospital medicine* (pp. 213–229). Philadelphia: Lippincott Williams & Wilkins.

Hannon, D.W. & Steed, D.R. (2003). Specific congenital heart diseases. In R.M. Perkin, J.D. Swift, & D.A. Newton (Eds.), *Pediatric hospital medicine* (pp. 230–240). Philadelphia: Lippincott Williams & Wilkins.

Harlingue, A.E. & Durand, D.J. (2001). Recognition, stabilization, and transport of the high-risk newborn. In M.H. Klaus & A.A. Fanaroff (Eds.), *Care of the high-risk neonate* (5th ed., pp. 65–99). Philadelphia: W.B. Saunders.

Hulett, L.L. & Ovitt, T.W. (2001). History and physical examination. In H.D. Allen, H.P. Gutgesell, E.B. Clark & D.J. Driscoll (Eds.), *Moss and Adams' heart disease in infants, children, and adolescents* (6th ed., pp. 162–170). Philadelphia: Lippincott Williams & Wilkins.

Johnson, J.J. (1999). Plethora and pallor. In P.J. Thureen, J. Deacon, P. O'Neill, & J. Hernandez (Eds.), *Assessment and care of the well newborn* (pp. 261–266). Philadelphia: W.B. Saunders.

Johnson, W.H. Jr. & Moller, J.H. (2001). *Pediatric cardiology.* Philadelphia: Lippincott Williams & Wilkins.

Jones, C.H. & Gawronski, M.J. (2002). The genetics of 22q11.2 deletion syndrome. *Progress in Pediatric Cardiology.* 15, 99–101.

Kliegman, R.M. (2001). Problems in metabolic adaptation: Glucose, calcium, and magnesium. In M.H. Klaus & A.A. Fanaroff (Eds.), *Care of the high-risk neonate* (5th ed., pp. 301–323). Philadelphia: W.B. Saunders.

Kourembanas, S. (1998). Shock. In J.P. Cloherty & A.R. Stark (Eds.), *Manual of neonatal care* (4th ed., pp. 171–173). Philadelphia: Lippincott-Raven.

Lister, G. & Apkon, M. (2001). Circulatory shock. In H.D. Allen, H.P. Gutgesell, E.B. Clark & D.J. Driscoll (Eds.), *Moss and Adams' heart disease in infants, children, and adolescents* (6th ed., pp. 1413–1431). Philadelphia: Lippincott Williams & Wilkins.

Lott, J.W. (2003). Assessment and management of the cardiovascular system. In C. Kenner & J.W. Lott (Eds.), *Comprehensive neonatal nursing* (3rd ed., pp. 376–408). Philadelphia: Saunders.

MacLellan-Tobert, S.G. & Porter C.J. (1998). Ebstein's anomaly of the tricuspid valve. In A. Garson, Jr., J. T. Bricker, D.J. Fisher & S.R. Neish (Eds.), *The science and practice of pediatric cardiology* (2nd ed., pp. 1303–1315). Baltimore: Williams & Wilkins.

Mair, D.D., Edwards, W.D., Julsrud, P.R., Seward, J.B., Danielson, G.K. & Goldmuntz, E. (2001). Truncus arteriosus. In H.D. Allen, H.P. Gutgesell, E.B. Clark & D.J. Driscoll (Eds.), *Moss and Adams' heart disease in infants, children, and adolescents* (6th ed., pp. 910–923). Philadelphia: Lippincott Williams & Wilkins.

Marino, B.S., Bird, G.L., & Wernovsky, G. (1999). Diagnosis and management of the newborn with suspected congenital heart disease. *Clinics in Perinatology.* 28 (1), 91–136.

Martin, R.J., Sosenko, Il & Bancalari, E. (2001). Respiratory problems. In M.H. Klaus & A.A. Fanaroff (Eds.), *Care of the high-risk neonate* (5th ed., pp. 243–276). Philadelphia: W.B. Saunders.

McGowan, J.E., Hagedorn, M.I.E., & Hay W.W., Jr. (2002). Glucose homeostasis. In G.B. Merenstein & S.L. Gardner (Eds.), *Handbook of neonatal intensive care* (5th ed., pp. 298–313). St. Louis: Mosby.

Meerstadt, P.W.D. & Gyll, C. (1994). *Manual of neonatal emergency x-ray interpretation.* London: W.B. Saunders.

Meliones, J.N. & Cheifetz, I.M. (1998). Pulmonary physiology and heart-lung interactions. In A. Garson, Jr., J. T. Bricker, D.J. Fisher & S.R. Neish (Eds.), *The science and practice of pediatric cardiology* (2nd ed., pp. 297–312). Baltimore: Williams & Wilkins.

Merle, C. (2001). Nursing considerations of the neonate with congenital heart disease. *Clinics in Perinatology, 28* (1), 223–233.

References

Minino, A.M., Arias, E., Kochanek, K.D., Murphy, S.L., & Smith, B.L. (2002). Deaths: Final data for 2000. *National vital statistics reports,* Vol. 50, No. 15. Hyattsville, MD: National Center for Health Statistics.

Moniaci, V.K. & Moniaci, S.D. (2003). Monitoring neonatal biophysical parameters in a developmentally supportive environment. In C. Kenner & J.W. Lott (Eds.), *Comprehensive neonatal nursing* (3rd ed., pp. 285–307). Philadelphia: Saunders.

Montoya, K.D., & Washington R.L. (2002). Cardiovascular diseases and surgical interventions. In G.B. Merenstein & S.L. Gardner (Eds.), *Handbook of neonatal intensive care* (5th ed., pp. 576–608). St. Louis: Mosby.

Morriss, M.J.H. & McNamara, D.G. (1998). Coarctation of the aorta and interrupted aortic arch. In A. Garson, Jr., J. T. Bricker, D.J. Fisher & S.R. Neish (Eds.), *The science and practice of pediatric cardiology* (2nd ed., pp. 1317–1346). Baltimore: Williams & Wilkins.

Mullins, C.E. & Pagotto, L. (1998). Patent ductus arteriosus. In A. Garson, Jr., J. T. Bricker, D.J. Fisher & S.R. Neish (Eds.), *The science and practice of pediatric cardiology* (2nd ed., pp. 1181–1197). Baltimore: Williams & Wilkins.

Neches, W.H., Park, S.C. & Ettedgui, J.A. (1998). Tetralogy of Fallot and tetralogy of Fallot with pulmonary atresia. In A. Garson, Jr., J. T. Bricker, D.J. Fisher & S.R. Neish (Eds.), *The science and practice of pediatric cardiology* (2nd ed., pp. 1383–1411). Baltimore: Williams & Wilkins.

Neches, W.H., Park, S.C. & Ettedgui, J.A. (1998). Transposition of the great arteries. In A. Garson, Jr., J. T. Bricker, D.J. Fisher & S.R. Neish (Eds.), *The science and practice of pediatric cardiology* (2nd ed., pp. 1463–1503). Baltimore: Williams & Wilkins.

Neish, S.R. (1998). Systemic blood flow and oxygen delivery. In A. Garson, Jr., J. T. Bricker, D.J. Fisher & S.R. Neish (Eds.), *The science and practice of pediatric cardiology* (2nd ed., pp. 231–240). Baltimore: Williams & Wilkins.

Novotny, W.E., & Perkin, R.M. (2003). Shock. In R.M. Perkin, J.D. Swift, & D.A. Newton (Eds.), *Pediatric hospital medicine* (pp. 199–208). Philadelphia: Lippincott Williams & Wilkins.

O'Leary, P.W., Mair, D.D., Edwards, W.D., Julsrud, P.R., Puga, F.J., & Goldmuntz, E. (2001). Pulmonary atresia and ventricular septal defect. In H.D. Allen, H.P. Gutgesell, E.B. Clark & D.J. Driscoll (Eds.), *Moss and Adams' heart disease in infants, children, and adolescents* (6th ed., pp. 864–879). Philadelphia: Lippincott Williams & Wilkins.

Pagotto, L.T., Hawkins, J.A., Tani, L.Y., Pollard, H. & Minich, L.L. (2002). Management of cardiac anomalies associated with velocardiofacial syndrome. *Progress in Pediatric Cardiology. 15,* 135–144.

Park, M.K. (Ed.). (2002). *Pediatric cardiology for practitioners* (4th ed., pp.3–33, 52–59, 67–77, 87, 93–97, 106–112, 113–126; 155–173, 174–185; 189–194, 196–199, 202–240, 247–251, 256, 261, 333–348, 349–351, 365–371, 372–396, 417–426, 471, 489, 498, 501). St. Louis: Mosby.

Parry, W.H., & Zimmer, J. (2002). Acid-base homeostasis and oxygenation. In G.B. Merenstein & S.L. Gardner (Eds.), *Handbook of neonatal intensive care* (5th ed., pp. 179–190). St. Louis: Mosby.

Perkin, R.M. & Steed, R.D. (2003). Cyanosis. In R.M. Perkin, J.D. Swift, & D.A. Newton (Eds.), *Pediatric hospital medicine* (pp. 109–115). Philadelphia: Lippincott Williams & Wilkins.

Perkin, R.M. & Swift, J.D. (2003). Intraosseous access and infusion. In R.M. Perkin, J.D. Swift, & D.A. Newton (Eds.), *Pediatric hospital medicine* (pp. 859–862). Philadelphia: Lippincott Williams & Wilkins.

Perry, J.C. (1998). Supraventricular tachycardia. In A. Garson, Jr., J. T. Bricker, D.J. Fisher & S.R. Neish (Eds.), *The science and practice of pediatric cardiology* (2nd ed., pp. 2059–2101). Baltimore: Williams & Wilkins.

Reddy, V.M., Underleider, R.M. & Hanley, F.L. (1998). Pulmonary valve atresia with intact ventricular septum. In A. Garson, Jr., J. T. Bricker, D.J. Fisher & S.R. Neish (Eds.), *The science and practice of pediatric cardiology* (2nd ed., pp. 1563–1577). Baltimore: Williams & Wilkins.

Rosenthal, G. (1998). Prevalence of congenital heart disease. In A. Garson, Jr., J. T. Bricker, D.J. Fisher & S.R. Neish (Eds.), *The science and practice of pediatric cardiology* (2nd ed., pp. 1083–1105). Baltimore: Williams & Wilkins.

Siegel, R., Gardner, S.L., & Merenstein G.B. (2002). Families in crisis: Theoretic and practical considerations. In G.B. Merenstein & S.L. Gardner (Eds.), *Handbook of neonatal intensive care* (5th ed., pp. 725–753). St. Louis: Mosby.

Singleton, E.B. & Morriss, M.J.H. (1998). Plain radiographic diagnosis of congenital heart disease. In A. Garson, Jr., J. T. Bricker, D.J. Fisher & S.R. Neish (Eds.), *The science and practice of pediatric cardiology* (2nd ed., pp. 715–734). Baltimore: Williams & Wilkins.

Simmons, R. (2001). Neonatal hypoglycemia. In R.A. Polin, M.C. Yoder & F.D. Burg (Eds.), *Workbook in practical neonatology* (3rd ed., pp. 63–70). Philadelphia: W.B. Saunders.

References

Siwik, E.S., Patel, C.R., Zahka, K.G., & Goldmuntz, E. (2001). Tetralogy of Fallot. In H.D. Allen, H.P. Gutgesell, E.B. Clark & D.J. Driscoll (Eds.), *Moss and Adams' heart disease in infants, children, and adolescents* (6th ed., pp. 880–902). Philadelphia: Lippincott Williams & Wilkins.

Southgate, W.M., & Pittard, W.B., III. (2001). Classification and physical examination of the newborn infant. In M.H. Klaus & A.A. Fanaroff (Eds.), *Care of the high-risk neonate* (5th ed., pp. 100–129). Philadelphia: W.B. Saunders.

Spilman, L.J. & Furdon, S.A. (1998). Recognition, understanding, and current management of cardiac lesions with decreased pulmonary blood flow. *Neonatal Network. 17*(4), 7–18.

Spoon, J.M. (2001). Situs inversus totalis. *Neonatal Network. 20*(1), 59–63.

Swinford, R.D., Bonilla-Filix, M., Cerda, R.D., & Portman, R.J. (2002). Neonatal nephrology. In G.B. Merenstein & S.L. Gardner (Eds.), *Handbook of neonatal intensive care* (5th ed., pp. 609–643). St. Louis: Mosby.

Sullivan, K.E. (2002). Immunologic issues in VCFS / chromosome 22q11.2 deletion syndrome. *Progress in Pediatric Cardiology. 15*, 103–108.

Taketomo, C.K., Hodding, J.H. & Kraus, D.M. (1998). *Pediatric dosage handbook* (5th ed.). Hudson, OH: Lexi-comp Inc.

Tappero, E.P. & Honeyfield, M.E. (2003). *Physical assessment of the newborn* (4th ed.). Santa Rosa, CA: NICU, Inc.

Townsend, S.F. (1999). Approach to the infant at risk for hypoglycemia. In P.J. Thureen, J. Deacon, P. O'Neill, & J. Hernandez (Eds.), *Assessment and care of the well newborn* (pp. 267–271). Philadelphia: W.B. Saunders.

Townsend, S.F. (1999). The large-for-gestational-age and the small-for-gestational-age infant. In P.J. Thureen, J. Deacon, P. O'Neill, & J. Hernandez (Eds.), *Assessment and care of the well newborn* (pp. 272–283). Philadelphia: W.B. Saunders.

Versmold, H.T., Kitterman, J.A., Roderic, Gregory, G.A., & Tooley, W.H. (1981). Aortic blood pressure during the first 12 hours of life in infants with birth weight 610 – 4220 grams. *Pediatrics, 67*(5), 607–612.

Waldman, J.D., & Wernly, J.A. (1999). Cyanotic congenital heart disease with decreased pulmonary blood flow in children. *Pediatric Clinics of North America, 46* (2), 385–404.

Ward, K.E. & Mullins, C.E. (1998). Anomalous pulmonary venous connections, pulmonary vein stenosis, and atresia of the common pulmonary vein. In A. Garson, Jr., J. T. Bricker, D.J. Fisher & S.R. Neish (Eds.), *The science and practice of pediatric cardiology* (2nd ed., pp. 1431–1461). Baltimore: Williams & Wilkins.

Wechsler, S.B., & Wernovsky, G. (1998). Cardiac disorders. In J.P. Cloherty & A.R. Stark (Eds.), *Manual of neonatal care* (4th ed., pp. 393–451). Philadelphia: Lippincott-Raven.

Wernovsky, G. (2001). Transposition of the great arteries. In H.D. Allen, H.P. Gutgesell, E.B. Clark & D.J. Driscoll (Eds.), *Moss and Adams' heart disease in infants, children, and adolescents* (6th ed., pp. 1027–1084). Philadelphia: Lippincott Williams & Wilkins.

West, J.B. (1990). *Respiratory physiology – the essentials* (4th ed., pp. 69–85). Baltimore: Williams & Wilkins.

Witt, C. (1998). Cyanotic heart lesions with increased pulmonary blood flow. *Neonatal Network. 17*(7); 7–16.

Yager, J.Y. (2002). Hypoglycemic injury to the immature brain. *Clinics in Perinatology. 29* (4), 651–674.